THE NEW JOY OF
GAY SEX

THE NEW JOY OF GAY SEX

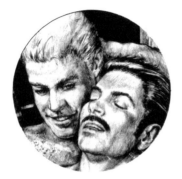

DR. CHARLES SILVERSTEIN
AND FELICE PICANO

PREFACE BY EDMUND WHITE

BLACK-AND-WHITE ILLUSTRATIONS BY
F. RONALD FOWLER

COLOR ILLUSTRATIONS BY
DENI PONTY

HarperPerennial
A Division of HarperCollins*Publishers*

DESIGNED BY JOEL AVIROM

The Library of Congress has catalogued the hardcover edition as follows:

Silverstein, Charles.
The new Joy of gay sex / Charles Silverstein and Felice Picano. — 1st ed.
p.   cm.
New ed. of: The Joy of gay sex / Charles Silverstein & Edmund White. 1977.
Includes index.
ISBN 0-06-016813-7
1. Homosexuality, Male.   2. Sex instruction for gay men.
I. Picano, Felice, 1944–   .   II. Silverstein, Charles. Joy of gay sex.   III. Title.
HQ76.S533   1992
613.9′6 086642—dc20   92-52594

ISBN 0-06-092438-1 (pbk.)

97 DT/HR 10 9 8 7

To William (again), from Charles
To Will and David, and the younger generation, from Felice

CONTENTS

ACKNOWLEDGMENTS   x
PREFACE   xi
INTRODUCTION   xiii

LIST OF ENTRIES

AIDS (see HIV DISEASE)
ANUS   1
BARS   1
BATHS   2
BEAUTIES   3
BISEXUALITY   4
BLOW JOB   8
BODY FLUIDS   11
BODY IMAGE   11
BODY POSITIVE   12
BONDAGE   15
BOOZE AND HIGHS   16
BOTTOM   18
BOTTOMS UP   20
BUNS   21
CAMPING   23
CELIBACY   25
CIVIL RIGHTS   26
CLUBS   27
COCK SIZE   30
COMING OUT   32
COMPUTER SEX   36
CONDOMS   38
COUPLES   41
CRUISING   45
DADDY-SON FANTASIES   48
DANGEROUS SEX   50
DEPRESSION   53
DIRTY TALK   54
DOGGY STYLE   55
DOMESTIC VIOLENCE   56
DRUGS   57

EARLY ABUSE 59
EFFEMINACY 61
FACE-TO-FACE 61
FETISH 64
FIDELITY AND MONOGAMY 65
FINDING A PHYSICIAN 66
FIRST TIME 67
FISTING 71
FORESKIN 72
FRIENDSHIP 74
FROTTAGE 74
FUCK BUDDIES 76
GAY LIBERATION 78
GAY POLITICS AND POLITICIANS 80
GROWING OLDER 83
GUILT 84
GYMS 86
HAIR 87
HANDS 88
HIV DISEASE 89
HOMOPHOBIA 94
HUSTLERS 96
IMPOTENCE 97
INSURANCE 101
JEALOUSY, ENVY, AND POSSESSIVENESS 103
J.O. BUDDIES 105
J.O. CLUBS 106
KISSING 107
LETTING GO 109
LIVING WILLS 111
LONELINESS 112
LUBRICANTS 114
MARRIED MEN 115
MASSAGE 117
MASTURBATION AND FANTASY 119
MIRRORS 123
MIXED HIV COUPLES 124
MYTHIC BEGINNINGS 125
NEW MACHO IMAGES 128
NIBBLING AND BITING 131
NIPPLES 132
NOISEMAKING 134
ORGIES 135
PARENTS 137
PHONE SEX 139
PIERCING 142
PLEASURE TRAP 145
PORNOGRAPHY 146
PROBLEMS OF EJACULATION 148
PROMISCUITY 150
RACISM 152
RAPE 153
REJECTION 155

RELAXATION   156
RIMMING   156
ROLE-PLAYING   157
SADOMASOCHISM   158
SAFE SEX   161
SAYING NO   163
SCAT   164
SEDUCTION   165
SEX ADS   167
SEX CLUBS   168
SEX TOYS   169
SEX WITH ANIMALS   170
SEXUALLY TRANSMITTED DISEASES   172
SHAVING   178
SIDE BY SIDE   179
SIT ON MY FACE   180
SITTING ON IT   181
SIXTY-NINING   183
SLEAZY SEX   184
SPANKING   186
STAND AND DELIVER   187
SUICIDE   188
TEAROOMS AND BACK ROOMS   189
TEENAGERS   191
TENDERNESS   194
THREE-WAYS   195
TOP   197
TOUCHING AND HOLDING   199
TRADE   202
TRANSVESTITES AND TRANSSEXUALS   202
TRICKING   205
TYPES   207
VANILLA SEX   208
WATER SPORTS   210
WILLS   212
WRESTLING   214

INDEX   215

ACKNOWLEDGMENTS

Many people assisted us in the preparation of this book. Danny Neudell, a longtime friend, wrote a handful of essays for us. We received technical advice about STDs and HIV Disease from Dan William, M.D.; about legal issues and insurance from Carol Buell, Esq., Mark Scherzer, Esq., and Wendy Frank; about accounting from Buddy Dikman, C.P.A.; and about addiction from Mel Poll, M.D. John Ferrari, Gene Mendez, Al Sbordone, M.S.W., Ellen Ratner, M.S., Michael Shernoff, M.S.W., and Richard Walker contributed information and advice. Also Bree Scott-Hartland and members of the People with AIDS Coalition, the Education Committee of Gay Men's Health Crisis, and the House of Africa (Tracy Norman, Eddie Smith, and "Big" Kevin). The full manuscript was reviewed by David Drane, Terry Helbing, Keith Kahla, Keith McDermott, Will Meyerhofer, Meyer Morgenstern, Virginia Record, Mark Robinson, and David Sloan, all of whom tried to curb the excesses in our prose and fill the gaps in our knowledge. A special thanks to William Bory for his help.

PREFACE

The original *Joy of Gay Sex* was what was called in the business a managed book—that is, one packaged by the publisher. Under this system the publisher chooses the writers and illustrators and instructs them step-by-step in the fulfillment of a concept that originated with the publisher. It's a bit like the old Hollywood studio system in which writers were contracted to turn "properties" into scenarios. I was one of twenty-some writers asked to submit sample entries to the English publishers who'd made a killing with *The Joy of Sex* and hoped to repeat their success in companion volumes for lesbians and gay men.

Since I was supporting my nephew at the time and was crippled with debts, I put my heart into my entries on kissing, fisting, and cock size. Imagine my surprise when I found I'd been chosen and would be teamed up with Dr. Charles Silverstein, a friend for years.

We had to turn out the book in a very short time—three months, I think it was, in the innocent spring of 1977. I wrote day and night about blow jobs and rimming, but no matter how horny I became I couldn't afford the time off actually to have sex. My situation seemed worthy of Tantalus—condemned to describe what one would have preferred to do.

Charles and I made a good team, I like to think. He had come out rather late and gone almost instantly into a relationship, so it was up to me to describe cruising in bars and baths. But he'd worked extensively as a psychotherapist and with sexual dysfunctions, and it was he who knew what techniques to recommend for dealing with impotence, premature ejaculation, and delayed ejaculation. We both loved men, but he was more tender and sensual and I more hard-core.

I kept wondering whether to sign my real name to the book, but of course I couldn't sign a pen name to a book that called for total honesty. In fact, I discovered that signing it was the most liberating act of my life, the first time I identified myself as a proud homosexual. At the time I was sort of whistling in the dark, but I was the first to be convinced by the cheerful, confident tone of our own words.

Charles and I both received some touching letters from readers—and some heartrending ones. The best one I received started: "Dear Sir, I am the sort of homosexual you disapprove of since I am still in the closet. I am twelve years old."

Of course, after 1981 both Charles and I wanted the book to be updated with AIDS information, but the original publishing house had been sold, the text had been "packaged" and "licensed" to various distributors, and no one answered our queries. When the book finally went out of print, the rights reverted to us, and Charles decided to bring out a new edition, partly in response to gay bookstores that reported it was the most requested out-of-print title.

I was under contract to do another book, but I was delighted when Charles linked up with Felice Picano, an old friend, a splendid writer and, as the publisher of the SeaHorse Press, one of the pioneers of gay publishing. He has brought to the new edition his earthy, no-holds-barred sense of humor, his elegant style, and his vast experience of gay life and love. "Baths," "Coming Out," and "Cruising" are just the first few entries that have been updated or extensively rewritten, while "Mixed-HIV Couples," "Piercing," and "Phone Sex" are some of the brand-new entries.

In recent years when friends have asked me to sign their copies of *The Joy of Gay Sex* I've written, "Use it for fun—and in good health." That's what I wish every new reader as well.

Edmund White
Paris, France
December 1991

INTRODUCTION

A sixteen-year-old entered the Greyhound Bus Terminal in Boston. He had heard that gay men met there, and wanted to meet one and learn how to have gay sex. He was a beginner at cruising, but he picked it up quickly and within a couple of hours he was lying next to a man in a hotel bed, after having the first sex of his life. "That man was wonderful," he said many years later. "He was so patient with me."

When they said good-bye, the man gave the boy some money. The youngster didn't understand why, and was, in fact, quite upset. He was terrified that his parents would find the money and ask embarrassing questions. He decided to get rid of the cash by placing it in an envelope and mailing it to the Boston Museum of Fine Arts.

A week later, he returned to the bus terminal, and at the end of the day he mailed another envelope to the museum. And the next, and the next, and so on. The museum officials never knew who sent them all those anonymous cash contributions.

Sitting around the dinner table one evening years later, Ed White and Charles Silverstein, the authors of this book's first edition, listened to this story told by a friend. They went on to discuss their own youthful fears and yearnings.

The authors of the first edition agreed that *The Joy of Gay Sex* should be the kind of book our friend needed when he was younger; the book would be the perfect companion, one that would inform, be permission-giving, and describe sex as accurately as possible. They obviously had to talk about coming out and lovers, but also about friendship, civil rights, rejection, loneliness, depression, and venereal diseases. In the end, the book contained more nonsexual essays than specifically sexual ones, and might better have been entitled *The Joy of Gay Life*.

In 1977 the straight world was not ready to accept an open celebration of gay sex, and the book encountered antisexual, homophobic resistance.

French customs had the book shredded; the British burned it. Although the book was translated into French and sold in Quebec, only a few smuggled copies circulated underground in Paris. No English publisher was brave enough to issue it in the United Kingdom.

There were many attempts to suppress it. The Winnipeg police raided a local bookstore on the complaint of a woman who claimed to have mistakenly picked up *The Joy of Gay Sex* thinking it was *Joy of Cooking*. She said she was shocked by the pictures. The affair was obviously a put-up job. The charges against the bookseller were dropped after a defense committee composed mostly of local college students publicized the actions of the police.

In Hamilton, Ontario, the book was removed from the McMaster University bookstore and transferred to the medical bookstore, as a result of a complaint by an anthropology professor who said of its illustrations: "I've never seen anything to equal them. They are definitely the most disgusting things I've seen on sale anywhere."

This sparked a heated controversy about free speech and censorship. The president of the university stepped in, announcing that moving the book "struck at the very nature of the university as a centre for free inquiry." He then ordered that it remain in the *medical* bookstore.

Canadian customs had seized a shipment of *The Joy of Gay Sex* because of its pictures and descriptions of anal intercourse. At the Toronto trial, Silverstein testified for the defendant, the Glad Day Bookshops. Her Majesty's Customs Officer maintained that pictures or descriptions of anal intercourse were prohibited. Under cross-examination, he asserted that a book's artistic, cultural, or educational value was "none of my business."

On March 20, 1987, Judge Ronald Hawkins ruled: "To write about homosexual practices without dealing with anal intercourse would be equivalent to writing a history of music and omitting Mozart."

Despite Judge Hawkins's decision, the Glad Day Bookshops continued to be harassed by customs authorities. Jearld Moldenhauer, owner of Glad Day Bookshops in Toronto and Boston, has been one of the unsung heroes in the fight against censorship. He stood alone, with little in the way of funds, against the might of the Canadian government.

In the United States, the book created a furor. At the time Anita Bryant was raging against homosexuality. Many bookstores, fearful of offending customers, kept the book out of sight. To buy it, you had specifically to ask for it. Nonetheless, some bookstores boldly carried the book and displayed it prominently.

The reaction of the gay community to *The Joy of Gay Sex* was electric. The information was pertinent, the tone just right, and the illustrations both sexy and accomplished. If *Joy* had been merely a pornographic book, it would probably have escaped the censors' notice, as so many pornographic books do: It would only have reaffirmed the prevailing heterosexual belief that gay life consists of sexual contacts but lacks love, affection, and the desire to build a caring community. *Joy* helped to instill pride and to encourage community-building in the gay world.

A little over a year ago, we were contacted by the owner of a bookstore in the Pacific Northwest. He was looking for copies of *The Joy of Gay Sex* and was surprised to find it was unavailable. Dismayed, he wrote: "This book shouldn't be out of print. People are coming out all the time. And especially now, more than ever, there's a real need for it."

More than ever. Since the first edition of *Joy*, AIDS (or HIV Disease) has become a terrifying fact of life. We had watched so many friends and colleagues die of this dreadful disease that we wondered if gays really wanted a revision of the book, or whether it would only serve as a reminder of the sadness and mourning that have afflicted the gay community since the early 1980s. We remembered the words of our friend Edmund White, who wrote: "It's just like the Middle Ages; every time you say goodbye to a friend, you fear it may be for the last time."

However, we realized, young gay men require updated information about safe sex practices—especially since the original version of the book was published in 1977, a time of few frank and detailed explanations of sexual practices and even fewer health concerns.

The current authors (Silverstein and Picano) discussed this revision with a great many people—writers, editors, doctors, and ordinary gays—then gauged their responses. We expected a variety of reactions from strong encouragement to outright disapproval. We were surprised when so many people enthusiastically urged us to put together a new edition, suggesting new topics. One consultant reminded us that with the original *Joy of Gay Sex* out of print, there was no longer a single, reliable guide to gay life.

Others pointed to the great changes in gay life since 1977: the rise of the new political activism, J.O. clubs, personal ads, and the astonishing growth of the phone sex business. AIDS has, of course, made it necessary to deal with many subjects once relatively unimportant: writing wills, buying insurance, testing HIV-positive, and talking to parents about being mortally ill. Our revision could bring together that new information and more.

On rereading the original volume we found attitudes about sex—indeed, about gay life itself—that now seemed excessively high-spirited, even rah-rah in their boosterism. Of course, we understood an ultra-positive attitude was necessary in 1977 when so much about gay life was terra incognita even to mature, experienced gays, not to mention young men just coming out. Strongly emphasizing the sunlight over the shadows had been a deliberate political act on our part. We therefore decided the new edition should be more pragmatic, and include essays on some unpleasant aspects of life, including racism, rape, and domestic violence. We also expanded the essay on dangerous sex. The new essay on parents reflects many gay individuals' experience that parents can be supportive or destructive toward gay sons. Safe sex guidelines are emphasized throughout the text. And we've tried to deal in an even-tempered, sometimes humorous way with lighter issues.

"Types" and "New Macho Images," for example, provide insight into prevailing gay attitudes and try to provide the texture of gay life as it is truly lived.

Some people, gay and straight, may be uncomfortable with the sexually permissive tone of this book. The book describes and illustrates a wide variety of sexual behaviors from "Vanilla" to "Sleazy." Inevitably, some of the essays about sex will be found to be offensive. "That's sick!" we hear gay men say about some aspect of someone else's sexual life—but not about their own. "Is there anything you guys are against?" might be one response to this book. Let's answer these criticisms now and be done with them. First, we are firmly opposed to censorship. We believe more harm comes from secrecy than from the dissemination of information, even if it is about the kinkier aspects of erotic life. We are also strongly against nonconsensual sex. Finally, we are not permissive about any dangerous or life-threatening form of sexual behavior. We state these dangers clearly and hope that men will make mature decisions. We believe strongly in safe sex guidelines and we provide information about them throughout the text. Except for these three limitations, we refuse to chastise people for their sexual fantasies and behavior. There's been far too much of that already. At the same time, we are not endorsing any specific sexual behavior. As Virgil said: *Trahit sua quemque voluptas* ("Each is led by his liking").

ANUS

Culturally induced fears have given many people phobias about their assholes. This bias against the anus is unreasonable. True, it is used for elimination, but so is the penis—yet that objection has not made the latter any less attractive. The anus is not only an avenue for elimination but also a sexual organ. It is highly sensitive, as it is lined with particularly responsive nerve endings. Moreover, the male anus is close to the prostate gland, and stimulation of the prostate is highly pleasurable.

All trace of shit can be banished if one takes the precaution of an enema before intercourse. Every drugstore sells disposable enemas or convenient bulb-shaped plastic enemas. (Daily use of enemas, however, should be avoided, as it could create psychological dependence and/or physical damage to the small intestine.)

People who are just beginning to experiment with anal sex sometimes fear that sticking a large cock up the anus will tear the skin; proper lubrication and relaxation, however, will prevent pain or damage (see *First Time*). More experienced men often worry that by repeatedly getting fucked they will lose the muscle tone in their assholes. There is no research on this problem, but it seems that many of these worries are unfounded and may act as a cover-up for feelings of guilt (see *Guilt*).

One occasionally finds gay men who disparage achieving sexual pleasure through their anuses. This might be a result of low self-esteem caused by the archaic notion that only women get fucked. This is both an insult to their own bodies and historically wrong, since men have found pleasure in their assholes since the time of the cavemen.

BARS

In a small town there may be only one gay bar. If you go to it, you're making an open declaration of your homosexuality. The straight townspeople may see you entering, and the gay clientele will immediately recognize you. The bar itself will probably be more chummy than sexual. There will be a regular crowd night after night, joking and socializing, and the atmosphere is likely to be warm, permissive, and lively.

In a big city, gay bars are far more numerous, anonymous, and specialized. A young dance crowd will go to one; older men will frequent another. In one, the latest fashions from Paris and Milan are on display; in another it's torn T-shirts, and crotch-gripping denims ripped at the knees, under the buttocks, and anywhere else deemed erotic; in a third it may be leather chaps, engineer boots, and black motorcycle jackets. There are also neighborhood bars somewhat like the ones in small towns. If you're just entering the bar scene or if you've just moved to a new city, you'll need to scout around. Local gay newspapers and the *Gayellow Pages* usually list bars.

There's not much to do in bars except play pool or pinball, drink, talk, and, in some cases, watch old movies, and dance. And, of course, cruise (see *Cruising*). Once you become known in a bar, people will probably gossip about you; you'll find you have a reputation, and even your sexual tastes will become common knowledge. Though this may strike you as intrusive, it does have a practical advantage: The men who do approach you are more likely to be compatible. If the typecasting becomes annoying, move on to a new bar (see *Types*).

If you're traveling, it pays to visit a gay bookstore first and buy an up-to-date bar guide. Visiting gay bars in other countries or communities is fascinating: It's the fastest way to learn different gay customs. One advantage to being gay is that no matter where you go you can establish an almost instant rapport with others like yourself.

BATHS

In the "good old days" (i.e., a decade ago) before the AIDS crisis, no visit to another city was complete without checking out its best-known "tubs"—Denver's Ball Park, Beverly Hills's Club 7009, and San Francisco's Ritch Street Baths were equivalents of the Rockies, the Hollywood sign, and the Golden Gate Bridge as must-see spots. Baths or bathhouses (known in Europe as saunas) were one of the most popular meeting places for gay men, and one of the few places where sexual contact was, if not guaranteed, then at least expected.

Which was pretty much their undoing. During the mid-eighties, political forces both within and outside of the gay community decided that bathhouses were loci of unsafe sex practices. Compromises were attempted in some cities: Literature about AIDS was strewn all over the bathhouses' public areas, and machines selling condoms and spermicidal lotions were placed next to those selling Dr Pepper and Sprite. In some cities, doors were removed from the rooms, and in San Francisco, "monitors" were appointed to rove the baths checking that people were not fucking, or sucking, without condoms.

But as the death toll from the disease rose dramatically, these half measures came to seem less attempts at preserving civil rights than a way of preserving a life-style—glamorized in the seventies—which seemed fatally outmoded.

Some gay bathhouses still do exist, and are, oddly enough, more prevalent in smaller cities than in larger ones, and mostly in the American South and Midwest and in Europe. (Although recently the few remaining in large cities have expanded as a result of increased popularity.) Lately they've been replaced by sex clubs. Should you happen to find yourself near a bathhouse, you may want to go in and at least look around. Lockers and rooms are usually available, the former often in a gymlike changing-room area. The rooms are usually small plasterboard cubicles containing a bed, a lamp, a tiny shelf, and nothing else. Bathhouse amenities generally include a pool or Jacuzzi that can hold anywhere from four to twelve people. Also likely are showers, saunas, and steam rooms; sometimes there's a dormitory area or a small gym or workout room; often there's a lounge with a TV or video screen for porno flicks or even old movies.

A night at a bathhouse can be a boring or an eye-opening experience. And who knows? You might even meet someone you like. If you have trouble insisting on safe sex, stay away. But if you decide to have sex, be certain it's safe sex. Even before the AIDS crisis, sexually transmitted diseases were a constant bathhouse problem. The same caution should be exercised in sex clubs (see *Saying No, Sex Clubs, Sexually Transmitted Diseases*).

BEAUTIES

A popular myth is that gay men go for "pretty boys." In fact, the range of gay taste is extremely complex and various, as is true of people in general, and tastes in looks change from decade to decade (see *Types*). Even so, there are absolute standards by which humankind has set apart those of outstanding physical attractiveness, and these criteria seem to last throughout the ages. It is this type of beauty we are addressing. If you happen to be a gay man possessing Apollonian beauty, you will already have been made aware of the fact. The special problems that beautiful men can have, precisely because of their beauty, are seldom discussed.

As everyone knows, a handsome gay man has the power to catch dozens of glances the moment he steps into a bar, strolls the beach, or arrives at a party. Sometimes it seems that doors—social, sexual, even career doors—magically open for him. What most people forget is that beauty can also inspire envy and nastiness. A handsome man enters a room. Someone desiring him but unsure of his own physical attractiveness or other good qualities may go through this thought process: "I want him; he'll never respond to me; who the hell does he think he is?" And the first words addressed to the handsome man are hostile.

Many are ready to dismiss a handsome man as shallow, stupid, or conceited; they concede his beauty but deny him other advantages. People also like to disparage someone very good-looking; beauties are often branded sluts or whores, though these words seldom make sense in what is, after all, an openly sexual situation. And should a beautiful gay man achieve fame, position, or wealth, it's often attributed to his looks alone.

Sometimes you may feel like saying, "I want to be loved for myself, not for my looks." But don't say it. Your looks are no more superficial than someone else's talent or wealth or celebrity—they gain you instant attention, and attract men.

Many beautiful men—gay and straight—are like the rest of us, uncertain of themselves despite their good looks. As a result, they are often shy and seldom exude the warm confidence that would naturally attract most people's better instincts. On the other hand, they generally attract and befriend one other male—a special friend, someone a bit less handsome but often acceptable enough, who stands between the beauty and the world. He acts as escort, chaperon, and host—effecting introductions, allowing an ambience of comfort and relaxation even in public, offering advice from his more normal perspective on which person may or may not be worth the beauty's knowing. It's a symbiotic relationship, of course: The friend gains status and entrée through his connection with the beauty, and often turns out to have a more active personal and sexual life than his friend.

Remember, beauty will gain you an introduction anywhere, but it will never hold anyone very long. Whereas an otherwise creative and loving life will sustain you when your beauty fades.

BISEXUALITY

Perhaps no word in the area of human behavior is used with such imprecision. First let's talk about what bisexuality doesn't mean.

In the classical culture of ancient Greece and Rome, many adult men were bisexual in that they were married to women and had adolescent boys as lovers. This arrangement was probably responsible for some of the great epic and lyric poetry of Hellenic times. There was always an age difference between the males, and the older man had to play the "active" and "masculine" role in intercourse. If he wanted to play the "passive" or "feminine" role (that is, if he wanted to be fucked), he became an object of ridicule. This kind of sexual arrangement is *pederasty* (sex with adolescents) and should not be confused with the sort of bisexuality we want to discuss.

Similarly, we are not talking about sex between men who are normally heterosexual but because of sexual deprivation (in prison, say) turn to one another. Nor would we call a man bisexual who has sex exclusively with men although he is capable of great emotional intimacy with women.

We do not subscribe to Freud's theory of bisexuality, that everyone is bisexual at birth but at a certain point is forced to *unconsciously* choose either heterosexuality or homosexuality. Freud, like many of his age and culture, believed that the only correct choice was heterosexuality.

Nor are we talking about the so-called bisexuality of closeted gay men. Many exclusively homosexual men pose as bisexuals, though they have sex only with other men. Their "bisexuality" is a convenient if dishonest passport into heterosexual respectability; it's often assumed for business or social reasons.

What, then, is a bisexual? A bisexual is someone who has sexual relationships with both sexes. A bisexual can have affairs with men and women

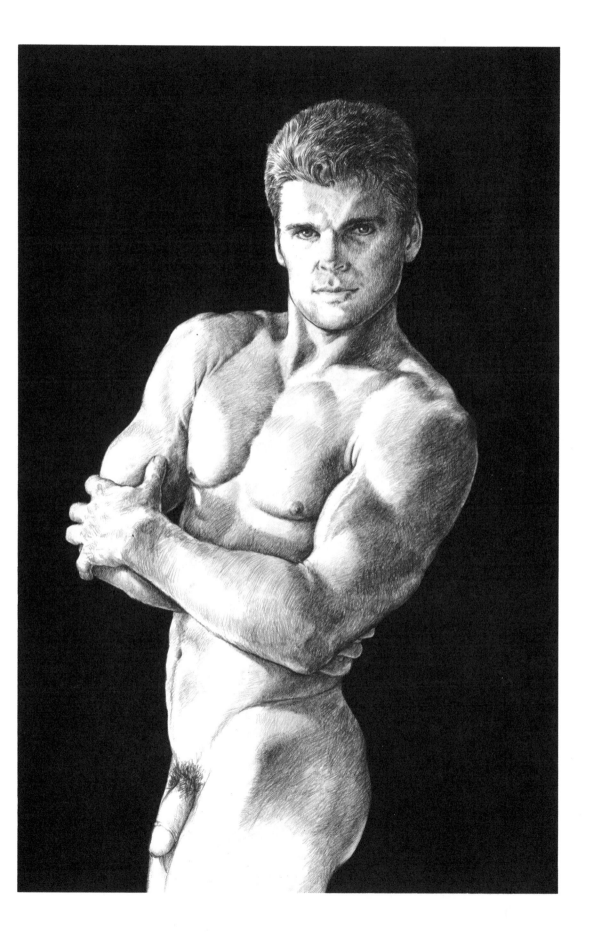

simultaneously, while other bisexuals have long homosexual affairs that may last for years; the bisexual will then enter into an equivalent long-term heterosexual relationship. Obviously these arrangements are fraught with complications.

One great advantage to bisexuality is that it enables someone to play very different emotional and sexual roles. With a woman, the bisexual might be fatherly and assertive, and with another man, childlike and passive. With a woman he might be open and cheerful and confiding, a true partner in a complex relationship, and with a man he might be impersonal, anonymous, and passionately animal. Or he might be tender and supportive with a younger man and rather rough and competitive with an older woman. Homosexuality might be reserved for lasting relationships and heterosexuality for occasional thrills, or vice versa.

The possibilities are various, and not all of them entail a clear separation between sexual and psychic response. Some bisexual men have arrived at a blend of the traits usually considered "masculine" and "feminine." They react to members of either sex in much the same way.

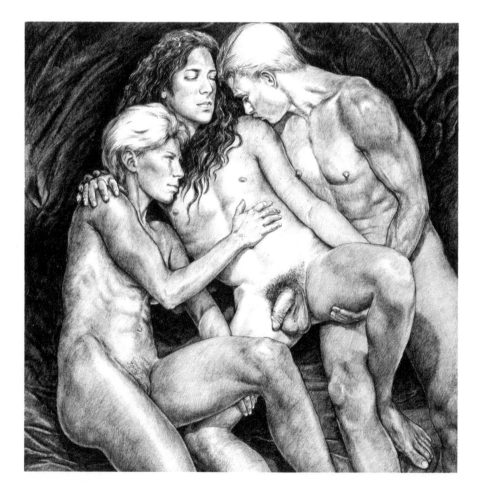

There are some problems in this polymorphous paradise. Truly bisexual men and women belong to one of the most persecuted groups in society. Both gays and straights find them confusing, and their very existence threatens widely held preconceptions. Many heterosexuals secretly believe that if a homosexual could know the joys of straight life he would be an instant convert. Conversely, many gay men consider their own lives so clearly superior to the "dullness" of heterosexuality that they ascribe bisexuality to hypocrisy or cowardice.

Gay life constitutes a genuine society complete with its own slang, humor, mating rituals, and gathering places—even, in larger cities, its own economy. Such ready-made institutions do not exist for bisexuals. They must carefully pick and choose among their straight and gay friends to shape a life tolerant of their catholic tastes.

For some men, bisexuality is simply a transitional stage between heterosexuality and homosexuality. The joke goes like this: A bisexual is a guy who is cuter than his date. Bisexuality can provide a resting place for assessing one's own inner feelings and values, and the reactions of one's friends and family. But if the pose is maintained too long it can become an act of bad faith, of self-deception, and a source of pain.

What if a man who has been happily homosexual for years finds himself attracted to a woman? Should he have an affair with her? If there is a real sexual attraction, why not? If you go to bed with her just a few times and make no promises. Should you tell her about your homosexuality? Most men won't, but then most men seldom talk about their past with women they have just met. But should you continue the affair, and if she begins to become involved, you should tell her. She may back out; she may try to "cure" you, in which case set her gently but firmly in place. If you're lucky, she may simply take you at face value and enjoy your relationship moment by moment.

What if you enter an affair with a man who has been heterosexual till now? From time to time straight men, especially if they are sophisticated and live in big cities, do develop a crush on a man they know to be gay (see *Straight Men*). If you find him attractive, there is no reason not to go ahead. But if you know his wife or steady woman friend, you may find yourself entering a romantic triangle not very different from an all-straight or all-gay one. Be prepared to lose both his friendship and hers.

Once you have your newly bisexual male in bed, you'll probably be surprised by how gentle he is. Many women train their male lovers to be tender and romantic, and the result can be something of a shock to a gay man entertaining fantasies about a tough, brutal straight guy. He may want you to fuck him or he may want to suck you off. He may not be good at either (after all, he's had no experience), but his secret reason for trying homosexuality may be to experiment in precisely these new areas. He might also be frosty with guilt the next time you meet. Don't worry that you're "corrupting" him; he is going into this sexual encounter with his eyes wide open. But don't expect a lasting relationship, no matter how much fun he is in bed. The main rule in dealing with straight men is: Be discreet. They worry more about their reputations than a Spanish virgin.

BLOW JOB

At some point in almost every gay encounter someone will probably offer his partner a blow job. This is nothing more or less than sucking cock, not as foreplay, but as a complete sexual act, including orgasm. The blow job is naturally the preferred method for quickies or when there is a danger of discovery, but its attractions are by no means merely functional. As a prelude to anal intercourse, as the theme in the duet of soixante-neuf (see *Sixty-nining*), a good blow job (which despite its name does not require blowing) is the ideal technique.

Until recently, in many European countries, blow jobs were virtually unheard-of between men, considered demeaning—they were only performed by women, and usually only by prostitutes. In the older and more sophisticated civilizations of the East and in societies of Africa, Asia, and South America, blow jobs are acceptable for everyone regardless of gender. Cleopatra of Egypt, for instance, is reputed to have sucked off a hundred Roman noblemen in one night, and a thousand Roman soldiers back home, but this is probably exaggerated.

It's difficult to say how it happened, exactly, but the United States has become the blow-job capital of the world: Men from all over the world vacation here, often traveling across country to experience the superb technical prowess of American cocksuckers.

The blow job is also the preferred and sometimes the only method of sexual contact between gay men and supposedly straight or married men (see *Married Men; Straight Men*). Guys otherwise indifferent and even hostile to gay sex will, on occasion and in the right mood, eagerly look for or at least accept a blow job from a gay.

A good blow job should be a pleasure rather than a task. And it can be pleasurable for the one sucking as well as for the one being sucked. Few who have experienced the subtle yet complete control of another's body and pleasure through his cock, and the thrill of carefully guiding that cock and that man to sexual fulfillment, consider the experience "demeaning"— or "passive."

There are several technical points to remember. Without experience and practice, it may not be possible to take a cock—especially a large one —in your mouth for more than two or three strokes at a time without gagging. (The gag response is, by the way, least active in the morning.) The solution: Use your hand as an extension of your mouth. Start off with your mouth alone, being sure to open it wide enough so that your teeth won't accidentally scratch the cock's tender flesh. Produce as much saliva as

BODY FLUIDS

The HIV virus, medical authorities believe, is transmitted by "body fluids." The fluids in question are blood, semen, and saliva. It is absolutely certain that the HIV virus can be transmitted by blood. It is most commonly transmitted in gay men through ass-fucking. It is less certain to what extent semen (or pre-come) ingested via oral sex can transmit the virus. While there are only a handful of documented cases of men who claim to have been infected through oral sex, most authorities still advise a conservative approach to sucking cock, which means using a condom. Few medical authorities (if any) now believe that tongue-kissing can transmit the virus. Feces, not strictly a body fluid, are not implicated in HIV transmission, though they can transmit other sexual diseases. One should use caution in cleaning up any body fluid from a friend or lover who is HIV-positive or has AIDS. (See *Condoms; HIV Disease; Safe Sex; Sexually Transmitted Diseases*.)

BODY IMAGE

There's a character in *War and Peace* who never realizes how beautiful she is. Her most dazzling attribute is her glance, her wonderful spiritual eyes, but when she studies herself in the mirror her eyes go dead. She becomes rigid and disapproving—and she remains ignorant of what everyone else knows, that she is the woman with the beautiful eyes.

Many people fail to perceive their looks clearly. We all carry around in our heads a sketch, if not a finished painting, of how we appear, and too often the sketch is unflattering. Sometimes the sketch may be redrawn along more attractive lines if we've been cruised heavily in the streets. But the next time we're ignored or rejected, the sketch turns into a caricature.

Not everyone goes through these agonizing fluctuations in self-esteem about his body, but there's bound to be some correlation between the way people react to your body and the way you regard it. If everyone tells you you look terrific, you'll begin to believe them—at least until the next time you face a mirror or have to choose some clothes or decide whether to grow a mustache.

It's not bad to be affected by what others say, but it's terrible to be ruled by it. It's worth remembering that what you consider your worst feature may strike others as your best.

Men with poor body images convey a sense of insecurity to the people they meet. Their very insecurity is off-putting and their fear of being ugly self-fulfilling. A few use their poor body image almost deliberately to keep other men at a distance. The scenario goes like this: "I'm ugly; he couldn't possibly like me; no one could like me; therefore I needn't risk getting close to anyone." Quite neat, really, but an awful way to live.

A poor body image can be improved. One way to let the light of reality invade this murky business is simply to ask a friend or friendly acquaintance what he likes about your body. You will be surprised when your partner praises your small ears or the "butch" veins on the back of your hands (butch? your *hands?*) or the rivulet of hair running from your navel into your crotch—features you've never given two thoughts to, since all you can think about is your giant nose and your forlorn buns.

If there's someone you trust completely, you might ask him to join you in an experiment. Have him sit in a chair and look at you while you stand and study yourself in the mirror. Tell him all the things you like about yourself—your wry smile, your big eyes, your powerful neck, your skin color, even the chipped tooth that you secretly pride yourself on. Naturally this orgy of self-regard will embarrass you at first, but it *is* curative. You can look at yourself in the nude or clothed. If you don't want to do all this in front of someone else, do it alone, but make sure that you say the complimentary things about yourself out loud. Why this viva voce approach should make a difference is not certain, but it does work. Perhaps people need to hear positive things about themselves, and not just think them.

If you wish to do something to improve your body, do it. Swim, take up a new sport, join a gym. When you begin to show physical gains, show them off with more revealing clothing or by going to a pool or beach; give people a chance to tell you about yourself. All too often false modesty or anxiety causes us to cut off compliments. Attend to other aspects of your appearance—your clothes or your hair; change any part of you that will give other people and yourself a visible sign you're feeling better about yourself.

And don't let anyone put you down!

Our advice boils down to setting your own standards for your looks rather than submitting to the standards (either real or imagined) of others. You must begin by yourself. After that, the good feelings you radiate will be magnetic to other men.

BODY POSITIVE

t's startling how our sense of time changes according to life's circumstances. The meaning of the word "lifetime," for example, is relative. Under normal circumstances, the word suggests a long span of years. But to the gay man who has just learned he is *HIV-positive* (another term is *seropositive*), the future is uncertain. He hears a clock ticking, and this changes his perception of himself and of the people around him.

Men react in different ways upon learning that they are seropositive. There is almost always a severe initial shock, followed by the quite natural fear of dying. Some men fall into deep depression and hide from family and friends, a response that only causes further isolation (see *Depression*). Contrarily, others venture out into the world of anonymous sex, as if the repetitive spilling of semen were an offering to heartless gods who imposed this epidemic upon them. Or they may surrender to low self-esteem, saying: "If I weren't gay, I wouldn't have this disease." A number of men are relieved at the diagnosis because the previous uncertainty may have been so much more painful than the reality.

More and more seropositive gay men are taking charge of their lives in the face of HIV infection by learning about the disease and its potential treatments. An excellent way to do this is to join or form a support group with other seropositive men. This essay, "Body Positive," is named after one such group in New York City. The People with AIDS Coalition (PWAC) is the most important support group for those already symptomatic. The communal experience of these groups is invaluable. Through participation one learns that life (including being HIV-positive or symptomatic) is about learning to *live well*, not about preparing to die. Experienced group members help new ones to see themselves objectively and to cope with both irrational fears and realistic problems. Call your local gay organization to find out which support groups meet near your hometown.

For the person just aware of his seropositive status, there are some concrete questions to be faced. Perhaps the most commonly asked is "Should I tell a potential sex partner I'm HIV-positive?" This issue sparks controversy among gay men. Some say no. They believe (not without good reason) that a potential sex partner may become frightened and flee. Being rejected under those circumstances is yet another wound. Handling it is only made more difficult by the added burdens of declining self-esteem, feelings of limitation, and lack of understanding from friends and family. From the point of view of these HIV-positive people, as long as they practice safe sex, they do not feel obliged to tell an anonymous partner. While this may be so, even these people believe that a potential lover must be told after only a few dates.

Other gay men adamantly refuse to hide the fact that they are HIV-positive or symptomatic. They believe other people have a right to know. Fed up with having hidden their homosexuality in their early years, these men divulge their seropositive status to friends, potential lovers, and family. They accept the possibility of rejection. One man expressed the prevalent attitude: "If they want to back off, fuck them." But many recall how often they've heard "You, too?" Be advised that some states have made it a crime if you do not disclose your HIV-positive status to a sex partner.

Which brings us to another often-asked question. Do you need to practice safe sex if both you and your partner are HIV-positive? The answer is yes! Semen and saliva are means of transmission for herpes simplex, hepatitis, cytomegalovirus (CMV) and Epstein-Barr virus (EBV) (see *HIV Disease*). CMV and EBV become activated in the presence of HIV, and you do not want to either transmit them to your partner or become infected with them yourself. There are also other sexually transmitted diseases (STDs) not directly related to the human immunodeficiency virus that can still be passed between partners; syphilis, for example, can be transmitted by oral-genital contact, and it's harder to treat in the presence of HIV. For the health of both men, safe sex guidelines should be followed. Couples should discuss these issues with their physician. (See *Sexually Transmitted Diseases*.)

Some seropositive men wonder whether they can have sex at all. Of course you should, but safely (see *Safe Sex*). HIV seldom inhibits the libido, and there is no reason to curtail your sex life as long as you do not put the other person at risk. However, that places a special responsibility on HIV-positive men to keep informed about the latest research on transmission.

Every seropositive man wonders whether medication or other procedures will keep the virus dormant. Questions of treatment are beyond the scope of this book, in part because so many new drugs are in various stages of testing. See *HIV Disease* for a list of newsletters about HIV treatments.

How will friends and family react to the news? Some friends will be supportive in every way possible. Others, motivated by fear, may show an exaggerated concern about your health, always asking how you're feeling. A few friends will disappear. Don't be shy about letting friends know if you want the news treated in confidence or whether they can tell other friends.

Parents are as varied in their responses as friends are (see *Parents*). Most are poorly informed about HIV and its effects upon the body. Some will panic at the news while others may go out of their way to deny you could have the virus; some—to still their own fears—may even deny the very real potential for illness. Most parents have turned out to be compassionate and supportive even though feeling overwhelmed by the news. In some cases, men decide not to tell parents at all, or only if they become symptomatic—especially if they've not been in close contact with their family.

There are practical considerations to being seropositive, particularly if you have a lover. You need to sit down together and plan for the possibility of illness, for its expenses, and to prevent homophobic family members from interfering with your intentions if illness occurs (see *Insurance; Living Wills; Wills*).

How should you act if you learn that a good friend is HIV-positive? It's quite common—if completely irrational—to suddenly feel afraid of the disease and of being contaminated by your friend. Don't feel guilty about it. Recognize that the epidemic *is* something to be afraid of but that social contact is *not* a route of the virus's transmission. In other words, it's okay to feel afraid—then get over it. It's also normal to have terrible feelings of inadequacy when your friend discusses his seropositive status with you. You may not be aware of it, but in truth you do know what he needs from you—it's exactly what you'd want from a friend if you were HIV-positive: continuing, unconditional love and support. Your first instinct may be to pull away, but remember he needs you more now than ever before. Touch him so he won't feel like a leper; hug him so he'll feel loved; kiss him so he'll know you're not afraid of him. It will do as much for you as it does for him (see *Touching and Holding*).

Once your affection with your friend is reestablished and solidified, you'll need time together to explore what his seropositive status means for the two of you in the future. Try not to change the relationship dramatically. Participate in whatever activities you did beforehand. Don't discuss your friend's diagnosis unless he initiates the talk. Friends often want to give advice about treatment, such as which drugs or treatment to take, or what physician (or healer) to trust. Hard though it may be, don't criticize your HIV-positive friend's approach to treatment. If he asks your opinion, give it without belittling his own beliefs.

BONDAGE

B ondage always implies domination, but not necessarily S/M. Some men like the sweet agony of being tied up and then subjected to a long blow job to which they can respond only with groans; or to having their bodies licked and caressed until they're mad with pleasure; or to being fucked in the mouth or in the ass while they writhe, unable to do anything to stop the action.

Other men prefer being the dominator. They like nothing better than to handcuff their partners or tie them tightly to the bedpost to feel complete control over them; the form of domination can then be teasing, gentle, or rough.

When it is a part of S/M sex, bondage is an extreme dramatization of the master-slave relationship: The master is in such total control that obedience is no longer an issue. The thrill for the slave comes from his being completely dependent on the master (and the complete trust this dependence signifies).

What to use in bondage? Some people prefer softer ties—silk, satin, chamois, any material that is completely pleasurable to the touch. Others prefer leather thongs and wear them wrapped around their necks when they go out at night, as advertisement and inducement. Still others use anything handy—telephone and electrical wiring, bed sheets, towels, metal and plastic police restraints—just as long as it fits into the roles being played.

We assume that you've chosen someone trustworthy to tie you up. To do otherwise is to place yourself in a particularly dangerous position. For example, a friend of the authors was sitting at home one evening. His doorbell started ringing, and didn't stop. When he opened the door he found his next-door neighbor on his knees, naked, arms and legs bound by rope, and ringing the bell with his nose. After having sex, the trick left him bound and robbed him (see *Dangerous Sex*).

The "bondage scene" in gay life can get beyond sexuality and become pretty arcane at times. The famous Mineshaft in New York City used to

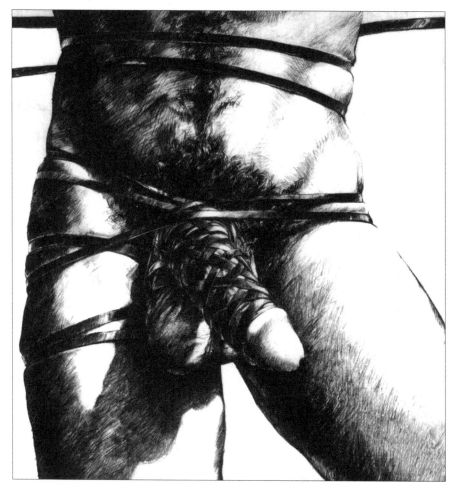

hold its Bondage Club's meetings on Sunday afternoons, and it wasn't surprising to walk in on a half-dozen young men trussed up by heavy hemp rope contorted into all sorts of positions, and to have a lecturer in full British Admiralty dress explaining the intricacies of the nineteenth-century English marine knots being used, a lecture that—save for the naked writhing bodies —might have been held in any museum, what with its precise terminology, wooden pointer, and avid listeners. (See *Piercing; Sadomasochism.*)

BOOZE AND HIGHS

Alcoholism and drug abuse are rampant in the gay community. There are many reasons why gay men subject themselves to the devastation of excessive drinking or the use of drugs such as cocaine, amphetamines, and barbiturates. By far the most important is the insidious effect of homophobia. For most of this century gay men could meet only in seedy, Mafia-owned, police-controlled bars in large cities, or furtively during late-night encounters in parks or woodlands, or in public toilets (tearooms). Gay men were forced to socialize in bars and around liquor, and since the bars opened their doors so late, they needed drugs to stay up at night. Gay men were always subject to capricious interrogation by police, to entrapment, and to seeing their names published in local newspapers under the headline PERVERTS ARRESTED. Little wonder gay men invariably felt ashamed of their sexual orientation and guilty over their sexual desires (see *Drugs; Homophobia; Guilt; Tearooms and Back Rooms*).

Drinking has always been used to lower social inhibitions. A drink or two gave a man more courage to ask another man to dance or for a date, and made rejection of the offer less painful. Repeated rejections often led to repeated drinks, or more drug-taking.

Feeling oneself a part of a special crowd of gay men is another reason some become dependent upon alcohol and drugs. Before they know it, they wake up one morning to discover they've traded their sense of inferiority and fear of rejection for acceptance among a group—along with an unwanted and unexpected chemical dependency.

Drinking and drug use continued over months or years can lead to abuse and addiction. The first stage of abuse is often hard to detect. Since your ostensible purpose in frequenting bars is to search for romance or sex, you will scarcely notice that your tricking has declined and your drinking increased.

Almost everyone drinks on occasion, and few gay men can claim to have lived a totally drug-free life. Experts generally call such people as those noted above drug *users*. Users do not have problems with chemical dependence. But the next category, drug *abusers*, includes those who, for instance, cannot perform sexually without alcohol or drugs or both. Drug abusers also suffer other adverse consequences, such as poor judgment in choosing sex partners, spending money capriciously, or falling down on the job. Drug *addiction* occurs when a person loses the power to make choices about his drinking and drug-taking. Chemical dependence becomes the tail that wags the dog. People who abuse drugs find that in time, the positive effects evaporate only to be replaced by negative consequences.

One important negative consequence is what experts call *disinhibition*. Most people feel inhibited and shy at times; alcohol and drugs remove inhibitions, making them feel bolder. But inhibitions (and caution) are sometimes appropriate to a given situation. Disinhibition gone awry leads to poor judgment. *Use of alcohol and drugs, for example, is the primary reason gay men practice unsafe sex.* This is true even of those who only use, rather than abuse, them. The disinhibition that results from alcohol or drug use also leads to other unsafe practices in which physical harm or illness may occur (see *Dangerous Sex; Fisting; HIV Disease*). Added to this is the fact that alcohol and drugs also further inhibit the immune system, and lead to a decline in T-cells. One would think these are enough reasons to be cautious about drug taking.

If you decide you have an abuse or addiction problem, you should join Alcoholics Anonymous or Narcotics Anonymous (listed in the phone book). If your lover or a family member has an addiction problem, join Al-Anon. Most large cities have gay AA (and Al-Anon) meetings. There you can meet other people who are seeking to escape drug dependence. Some people seek help through psychotherapy, which, in conjunction with AA, may be beneficial. Therapy alone, however, has not been very successful in dealing with alcoholism. Too many therapists regard alcoholism as a symptom of a neurotic disorder and will not treat the so-called symptom directly; and therapists cannot provide the round-the-clock support that most alcoholics need. (Read *Accepting Ourselves* by Sheppard Kominars.)

What if your boyfriend, best friend, or lover is an abuser? You may be in for a series of problems that may make you feel helpless and impotent to make changes. The first thing you'll learn is that you can't make him stop drinking or taking drugs. While you have every right to express your concerns, try to avoid blaming him or being self-righteous about the problem. Avoid increasing guilt, shame, or anger in your lover, and in yourself as well. But it's not possible to do this alone. You should join Al-Anon or Nar-Anon, organizations for people whose family members are alcoholics or drug takers. You'll find them listed in the phone book. That support may be vital for your self-esteem. Psychotherapy may also be useful.

BOTTOM

As you become more sexually experienced, you will soon discover your preferred sexual activities and positions. You may find that you prefer getting fucked, no matter the time, place, partner, or position. You may have also begun to find yourself evaluating the men you meet by a new index: the size, shape, and hardness of their cock, how much they check out guys' buns, and how often they come on by talking about fucking or saying they're interested in "getting ass."

When this happens you have become a *bottom*, or *bottom man*. The name, of course, derives from the placement of the person being fucked—i.e., on the bottom.

Being a bottom doesn't mean that you always have to fuck in the "missionary position." There are other positions (see *Bottoms Up; Face-to-Face*). Being a bottom doesn't make you less desirable than a top. It also doesn't mean that you're now only a bottom and can no longer do the fucking. Assuming you practice safe sex, feel free to fuck. Being known as a bottom can be useful in meeting potential sex partners, in that if your reputation precedes you, people not interested in being tops automatically eliminate themselves, while those interested in meeting bottoms may be interested when they weren't before. It's also useful when placing ads (see *Sex Ads*).

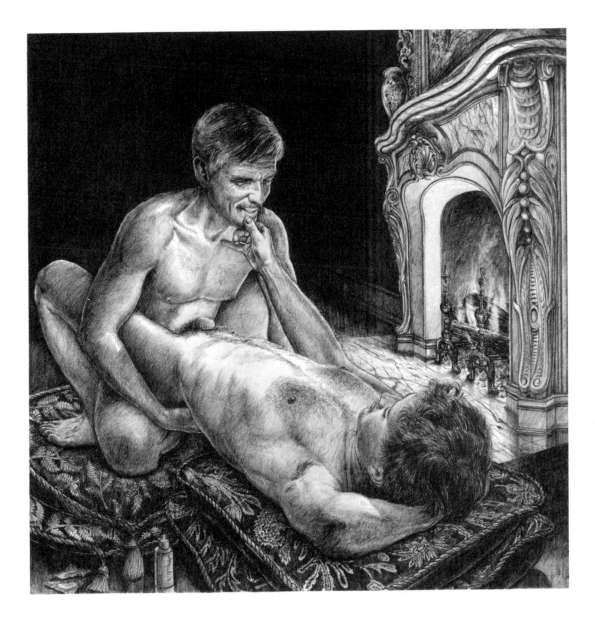

But we would be in error if we seemed to suggest that being a bottom is merely a matter of who fucks whom. It is, more importantly, a state of mind, a feeling one has about oneself in relationship to other men. "Bottom" (in sexual terms) denotes wanting to be taken care of and to be directed by the "top." In some men it may reflect an important streak of passivity, as if to say "I want to give myself up to you."

Psychologists have no idea how these preferences develop, nor how and why they change over time. It's probably best to indulge them as long as one makes decent choices in men, avoids heavy drugs and alcohol, and has safe sex (see *Booze and Highs; Drugs; Safe Sex; Top*).

Bottoms seem to predominate in gay life, although there are no studies to prove this. Quoting Mae West, bottoms are heard to say, "A good man is hard to find." The predominance of bottoms was demonstrated recently during "Underwear Night" in a South Miami club. Perhaps a thousand men checked their clothes and danced in their underwear. During the entertainment, the emcee, for reasons unknown, asked all bottoms to go to one side of the room and all tops to the other. Three-quarters were bottoms.

BOTTOMS UP

For the man turned on by the touch and sight of buns, nothing is more exciting than to see a partner lying on his stomach, legs spread apart, waiting to get fucked. In this position the shape of the buttocks seems rounder, their texture smoother and more cushiony. Sometimes when fucking someone who's lying on his back, you slam into nothing but hard bone and taut muscle (which, granted, can be a pleasure, too). But if your partner's on his belly, his buns are curved and supple and susceptible. A pillow under his pelvis will make his ass more prominent and adjust its angle.

Some men like to fuck guys draped over the broad arm or low back of a sofa or well-upholstered chair. Others like them standing against a wall, a window, even a mirror (see *Mirrors*), while still others prefer the classic simplicity of their lovers facedown, spread-eagled on a mattress.

For the man getting fucked, the very passivity of these positions can be a turn-on or a bore—it depends on one's mood and general sexual makeup. They're not very good positions for kissing or for watching the action or even for jerking off. You can reach around to steal an occasional sidelong kiss, you can watch yourself in a mirror, you can dry-hump the mattress or work your hand—or better yet, his—under you and beat off. But the real appeal of the position is its passivity.

For guys attuned to S/M, it can be the submissiveness of the slave. For the majority of gay men, the feeling of being covered and surrounded by another man can be comforting and secure. For everyone, the sense of being entered and massaged from within, over and over again, without any control, is primary, perhaps even primal.

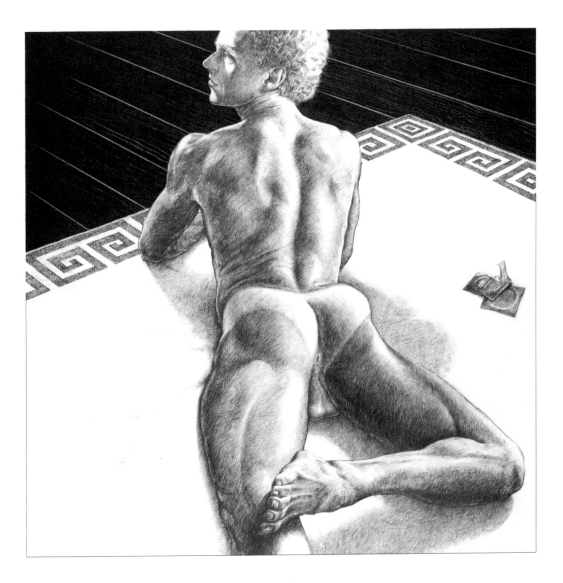

BUNS

They come in all shapes and sizes and there is an admirer for each variety. They are among the main attractions of the male body. Buns are versatile and beautiful—cushiony when relaxed, firm when flexed; at once soft and hard, smooth and strong, plush and steel. No wonder the world is filling up with replicas of Michelangelo's *David;* even in soapstone or Styrofoam, the rear view is beguiling. David's weight rests on one leg, which accentuates the roundness of that cheek and hollows out the dimple. The other curve is relaxed and the corresponding bun describes a gentler curve.

If jeans show off the ass, genes dictate its size and shape. There are many exercises for reducing but few exercises for building up the gluteus maximus, the largest buttock muscle; only those who do a lot of kicking (soccer players, swimmers, and dancers) are likely to improve noticeably on what God gave them. But there are a couple of exercises for transforming casaba melons into cantaloupes.

Stand upright. Step forward as far as possible with the right foot, bending the knee but keeping the torso straight. Your left leg will then be stretched out straight behind you; do not let the knee touch the floor. In one motion, push off with your right foot and return to a standing position. Repeat exercise, bending the left knee. Do three sets of twelve repetitions each. At first you will have trouble maintaining balance; hands on your hips will help, but practice will make perfect. After you have become used to the exercise and have done it for several days, do it with a light barbell on your shoulders.

Another exercise is this: Stand straight, holding on to a bar or shelf at hip height. Kick straight back with one leg as far back and as often as you can go. After you are sore, switch legs and do the same with the other leg. This tightens the bottom muscle and keeps the buttocks from sagging.

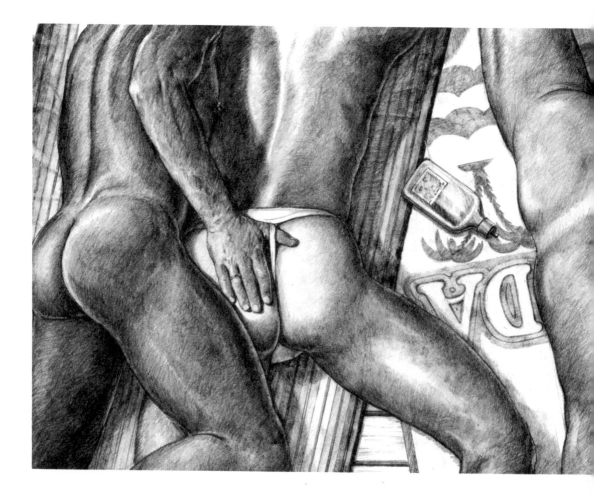

CAMPING

Camping is a form of pretense and humor that attributes—and then comments with much embroidering upon—effeminacy in a person or a group of people. Camp is opposed to seriousness, antithetical to tragedy, and represents the triumph of style over content. A bunch of gay men camping, for instance, can spend hours dishing one another (gossiping) and swapping insults (*"You're* secretly butch? Well, Mary, you'll die with that secret!"). In this guise camping tends to sound quite bitchy, even vicious, but outsiders often fail to pick up the fact that the insults being traded are all in good fun. During one such session, someone might say to another, "Miss Thing, you're the absolutely, drop-dead most vicious queen on this green earth!" and mean it as a great compliment.

Camping is a form of gay humor that is dying out. True, it may well have been the by-product of years of oppression, secrecy, and self-hatred, and now that gays are more self-accepting and somewhat less condemned by straight society they may have less of a need to camp. But the demise of

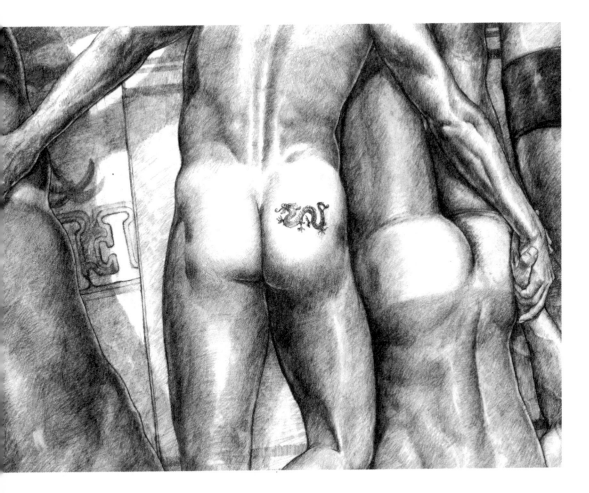

camp is not altogether a cause for celebration. Camping was and still can be terribly funny, and it does have one merit: It prevents gay men from becoming too pompous or serious in discussing their problems. One example of camp dialogue supposedly overheard during a police raid on the Trucks, a preliberation sexual gathering area in Greenwich Village: "Run, Mary! It's the cops!"—to which someone else responds, "Please, no names!" At its best, camp can be rebellious, elusive, dada, an anarchic force in gay life.

The word itself is odd; it may derive from army camp, where prostitutes —including male homosexuals—gathered. Or, it may come from "kemp," which in English dialect means "impetuous rogue."

Whatever its origins, "camp" is an extremely versatile word—a noun ("He's such a camp"), a verb ("Don't camp on me"), and an adjective ("His apartment is so camp: the interior of St. Lucy's, complete with confessionals!") As a noun "camp" means a funny, effeminate, or outrageous person or happening. As a verb it means "putting me on." The adjective signifies "amusing," even "preposterously amusing," and generally evokes a nostalgic interest in other periods, especially in bygone fads and follies.

Many women are insulted by the application of the feminine gender and exaggeratedly feminine qualities to men. This is understandable, but it misses the point. Camp seeks to disarm its enemies by identifying with the oppressors. If straight society accuses us of being women, we'll turn the accusation into a compliment. In fact, we will show them we're more outrageously feminine than they imagined. As blacks tease each other by calling themselves niggers, thereby defusing the insult hurled by whites, so gay men make a virtue out of the "vice" attributed to them.

During more repressive times, camp was the only way homosexuals could express their anger at a homophobic society. Their humor invariably mocked the hypocrisy and prejudice around them. Those men will be sorely missed.

Homosexuals eager to maintain a highly masculine image also object to camping, on the grounds that a conspicuous display of effeminacy only blackens the already tarnished picture straights have of gays. This objection seems misguided; bigots do not make distinctions between shades of effeminacy or masculinity. It's enough that you're gay for them to hate you.

Ever since 1964, when Susan Sontag wrote "Notes on Camp," "camp" has taken on another, more specialized sense. It's meant a sensibility peculiar to gay men fascinated by pop culture, by aging divas, failed movie stars, all the absurd pretensions of the past. This fascination, Sontag points out, is not cruel curiosity but an affectionate regard for "failed glamour."

> The experiences of Camp are based on the great discovery that the sensibility of high culture has no monopoly on refinement. Camp asserts that good taste is not simply good taste; there exists, indeed, a good taste of bad taste. . . . Camp taste is, above all, a mode of enjoyment, of appreciation—not judgment. Camp is generous. It wants to enjoy.

At least, that glamour conscious enough to be ironical about itself. Thus all the Tallulah Bankhead jokes. Example: The well-known actress with the deep voice is in a public john and notices there's no toilet paper. She asks for some from the occupant of the next booth, who reports she's used the last piece. Tallulah meditates, then replies: "Well then, darling, do you have two fives for a ten?"

CELIBACY

Celibacy simply means refraining from sexual activity, but over the centuries a great deal of fact, myth, and fallacy have attached themselves to the word and the practice. Those who are celibate because it is required by a religion or sect usually refrain from *any* sexual activity, including masturbation. In some religions—Catholicism, for example— even sexual thoughts are prohibited to the clergy. Nonreligious, less strict interpretations of celibacy do allow sexual thoughts, erotic fantasies, and daydreams along with masturbation, but do not admit sexual contact with another person.

But why, you might ask, would a sane person think of practicing celibacy?

The answer is that while it may be unusual for most adults, celibacy is not bad for you, either mentally or physically. The male body has a built-in method for ridding itself of semen (hence, nocturnal emissions) and in some cases celibacy can actually be refreshing. For example, gay men undergoing psychotherapy because of troubled romantic relationships often end them and avoid new ones so as to sort out their lives. One also finds celibacy as the choice of some men who are either HIV-positive or symptomatic (see *Body Positive; HIV Disease*). In these men, celibacy may be either the effect of depression or the fear of contaminating another.

What most discover when they become celibate is a surprising lack of pressure and stress in their lives. They feel relieved, relaxed, capable of being more objective about themselves and their relationships to others. Without the constant need to be sexually desirable, they begin to recognize abilities and values in themselves that may have been overlooked or underrated: charm, a sense of humor, psychological penetration, conversational ability, creativity. Work on these areas (free of sexual pressures) can lead to a fuller sense of yourself, providing a new confidence which ultimately makes you even more desirable should you decide to end your period of celibacy.

CIVIL RIGHTS

"What do these people want?" ask some uncomprehending heterosexuals about the civil-rights demands of gay liberationists. "The same things you have," we answer, "no more—no less!" In most of the states and cities of the United States, we gay people are not protected from discrimination. Whereas African-Americans, Latinos, Asians, and Jews face dreadful discrimination, they at least have the possibility of legal recourse. Gays, however, can seldom fight discrimination in the courts. Even the Supreme Court has declared our social identity illegitimate.

Civil rights is the most important issue in the gay liberation movement (see *Gay Liberation*). In almost every state, gay groups are lobbying for laws forbidding discrimination in employment and housing. Bigots have opposed equal-employment legislation, with the slander that gay firemen or policemen attempt to seduce their colleagues and that gay teachers corrupt their students. The fact that gays have been working in these occupations for years without creating such problems is conveniently ignored (see *Mythic Beginnings*). Fortunately, gay cops and firemen are coming out on the job and teaching their colleagues about homophobia.

Many states have repealed their sodomy laws, but in approximately half the states of the Union, such laws are still on the books. Although statutes vary greatly from state to state, they generally prohibit a number of sexual practices performed by either homosexual or heterosexual consenting adults in private. These illegal practices include anal intercourse and oral-genital sex. The same strictures that penalize homosexual sex also forbid a husband and wife to sixty-nine although the Supreme Court has stated that it might mind its own business about heterosexual sodomy, but still okay laws against homosexual sex.

Yet another area of gay legal struggle involves children in divorce cases. In the past, judges routinely refused to award custody to a gay parent and sometimes even forbade visiting rights to gay parents.

Gay couples want to adopt children, but the laws of many states prohibit it. Even so, thousands of children have been adopted into loving homes. Gay people want the opportunity to be judged worthy parents on the same basis as heterosexuals. (Read *A Legal Guide for Lesbian and Gay Couples* by Haydin Curry and Denis Clifford.)

Many people will be surprised to learn that a gay person may be prohibited from naming his or her lover as the beneficiary of a life-insurance policy. Insurance companies can also refuse a family medical policy to a gay couple and their children and insist that each member of the family take out a separate policy—an expensive procedure (see *Insurance; Wills*).

Domestic-partnership bills have been introduced in a few cities. San Francisco has a registration service for gay as well as unmarried straight couples who've lived together a certain number of years, signifying that they are "families" and are to be treated as such in housing, employment, and hospitalization. A number of cities, among them Boston, Seattle, New York, and West Hollywood, have established limited domestic-partnership rights for their municipal employees; other municipalities are slowly moving in the same direction. Many private companies have nondiscriminatory employment policies that protect gay couples.

AIDS discrimination is still severe everywhere. Many straight people fear that they or their families will contract the illness. Homophobic politicians pander to the hysteria and propose bills to place HIV-positive men in concentration camps. Seropositive men have been jailed for having sex even when safe sex guidelines were followed. Some states (Colorado for one) keep lists of people who are HIV-positive or symptomatic; but, gay liberationists ask, for what purpose? Contact tracing and mandatory HIV testing are viewed by gay liberationists as new tools in the hands of homophobes to discriminate against gay people, and by medical and social workers as virtually useless in hindering the spread of the disease. Oddly, at the same time that money is being spent on these panic-driven efforts, funds for education about the AIDS virus have been reduced.

Immigration authorities have the legal right to forbid entry into the United States to any person who is HIV-positive, and immigration laws against gays have not yet been completely removed. This would require an act of the U.S. Congress. Fortunately, homosexuality can no longer be cited as grounds for denying citizenship.

There have been gains and losses in the civil-rights struggle. The gains have come about because gay people became more militant in their demands, and more efficiently organized (see *Gay Politics and Politicians*). There is just as much need for militancy today as there was on the night of the Stonewall Riot of 1969, when transvestites attacked the cops, beating them to the ground with their purses and high heels. We believe that each of us owes a responsibility to those gay men who will follow us, a responsibility to make their lives a bit easier than our own.

One way to fulfill this responsibility is to join a gay-rights organization. It may be militantly political, or it may quietly serve the community. Some gay men think that such activity is truly the final stage of coming out. It is an enriching experience.

CLUBS

Your friends invite you out dancing at a club. It's probably not an all-gay club; possibly only Saturday or Sunday night is a "gay" or "all-men" night, while during the week the place caters to all comers. You pay at a booth, or hand in your complimentary tickets. The entrance may be up a long escalator past palm trees and mirrored walls, or down a twisting staircase into a neon extravaganza; or you may be whisked up in an elevator and when the doors part find yourself in a long corridor, pools

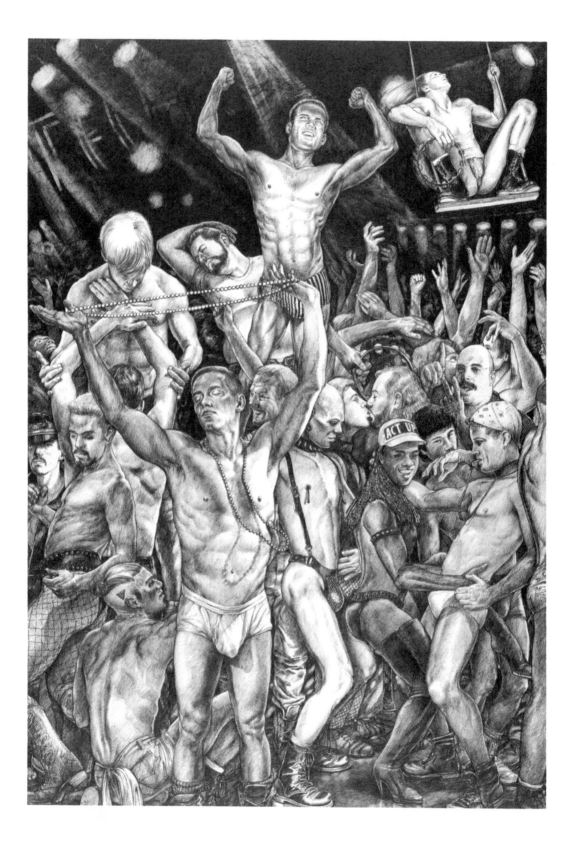

of light on the carpet. The main room is huge. Hundreds of men (and a few women) are on the dance floor, gyrating under a medley of shifting lights and booming sounds. The dancers seem to be mostly in groups; a few are in couples. When you and your group take to the floor, you affect a certain nonchalance, though actually you might be thrilled to be surrounded by so many different men.

After ten or a hundred songs have blended seamlessly into one another and you're quite exhausted, you desert your group and enter the refreshment room. Maybe alcoholic drinks are being served—or instead, Coke, ginger ale, and fruit juices—and there may also be snacks, piles of nuts and fruits to nibble on. An old movie is being projected against the wall, over and over again and without the sound. You sit down beside some perfect strangers, who smile and offer you a joint. Although they seem pleasant enough, you don't know them (or their level of drug usage) and you're already a little stunned from the music and exertion. Perhaps you only take one tiny hit, or you decline altogether. You want to enjoy yourself and experience everything. You return to the dance floor. Strobes are flashing; the speakers are belting out the latest hit; next thing you know your feet have a will of their own. Gay people, you decide in a burst of chauvinism, really are better dancers than straights.

There is no better proof of the emergence of gays from their closets than the continued existence of such clubs. Gays had no choice before gay liberation. They could only gather in sleazy hideaway bars buried in basements and as hard to gain admittance to as speakeasies. Now hundreds of gays troop into big, spacious, luxurious clubs where the dancing, the sounds, the lights, and the company are great. And when bars open that are reminiscent of the older kind, they usually make that resemblance a point of interest, calling themselves the Dungeon or the Firetrap. During the heyday of disco dancing in the late seventies, the main problem the gay clubs faced was how to keep straights from moving in and elbowing out the original gay clientele. At gay resorts and many urban centers, the favorite gay events are usually "tea dances," held in the afternoon and early evening on weekends, with fewer drugs, less drinking, but often the same good music.

A new generation is trying to retain most of the best aspects of the traditional older gay clubs, while updating them to meet their own needs and interests. Many newer clubs are smaller than the dance palaces of the past, far less glitzy, homier; they are located not in the usual gay ghettos, but in working-class, mixed, or ethnic neighborhoods. This reflects a desire both to strike out on their own and to be more politically aware. As a rule, the young men filling these clubs have particular interests in fashion, politics, and music (see *New Macho Images*). The latter ranges from the Metal Rock found in many slam-dance clubs, to rap, hiphop, and house music. Other clubs stress an interest in gender-bending and cross-dressing, with transvestite and performance artists.

In some large cities, the most attractive younger gays are now abandoning even those places to flock one or two nights a week to the local dance club savvy enough to offer entire nights of roller dancing. This quite traditional (your parents and grandparents went roller-skating) kind of event had a brief resurgence in the seventies and was boosted by the Broadway musical *Starlight Express;* it's been further reinvigorated by the appearance of the fast new single-blade skates, along with the colorful, muscle-revealing, eye-catching spandex, Lycra, and Velcro outfits favored by the street skaters you see flashing by.

COCK SIZE

What a tiresome obsession it's become! The man with a big cock feels that he is valued for his appendage alone. The man with a small cock is embarrassed by it and feels that he is spurned because of it. Size queens turn down a lot of sexy men because they fall a millimeter short of the desired length. Most men fear that their cocks are not large enough; the fear is often a cover-up for other insecurities.

Cocks vary greatly in length, width, and shape. Some are straight when erect; others curve back or sideways. A particular cock can also appear small when soft and surprisingly bigger when hard. Conversely, some cocks that are large when flaccid become only slightly longer when hard. But an obsession with size—your own or someone else's—only serves to reduce you or him to a statistic, and society is already too preoccupied with quantifying human beings.

At the end of the nineteenth century, a French physician, Dr. Jacobus (the nom de plume of Jacobus Sutor), actually made a survey of cock size in Africa. He was a French army surgeon assigned to various colonial outposts, where he conducted research. Part of that research was to run from village to village measuring the dick of any man who consented; it's unclear whether the French government authorized the project. Jacobus claimed that Sudanese Africans had the largest cocks, with Arabs running a close second. (He didn't measure those of the French soldiers in Africa.) The largest cock he encountered belonged to a Sudanese and measured 12 inches in length, with a *diameter* of 2¼ inches. "The unfortunate Negro who possessed this 'spike,' " said Dr. Jacobus, "was an object of terror to all the feminine sex."

If you think your cock is too small, don't fuss with vacuum pumps or hormones or other contraptions, because they don't work for enlargement —although they have other uses (see *Sex Toys*). Nor should you pad your crotch; false advertising will hardly make you feel more secure.

What you can do is to realize that your cock has many other aspects than size alone. A lover or fuck buddy can give you feedback—you may be surprised to learn he likes the way it curves up when hard or the way that

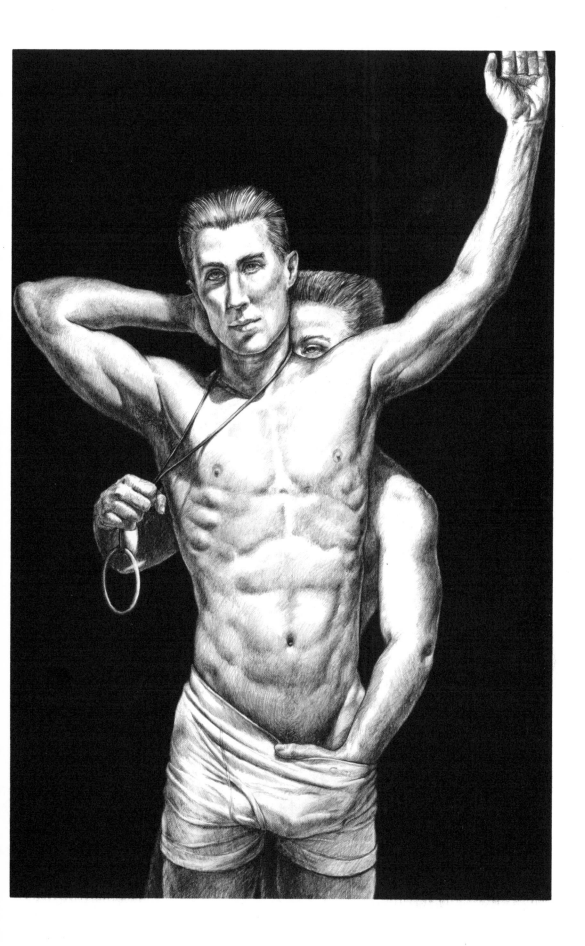

large blue vein zigzags down its length; he may like it just because it's fat and stubby. He may think that your cock is in perfect proportion to the rest of you; he may be glad your cock is no bigger than his. You are probably aware of the various attractions of other men's cocks, but in contemplating your own you may make the mistake of seeing its size alone. If you like another man's cock, be sure to tell him about it; he, too, needs reassurance.

(See *Foreskin*.)

COMING OUT

Coming out is not just the first time one has sex with another man. It is also the adoption of a psychological and social stance and it is the public stance that we take toward our homosexuality. In the past, few people were lucky enough to have come out in a relaxed way. Perhaps today fantasy and reality can come a little closer:

You've gone to the far end of the beach (where you know men in pairs and groups hang out) just because . . . well, just for fun. You don't really give it much thought, wanting to sun with these guys, but you do notice your mounting excitement. They all seem to be having fun. In the water two slender fellows are sitting on the shoulders of beefier guys and playing war. Near you another group, all well built and methodically tanned, are playing cards on a blanket and listening to a radio.

Right next to you is a tall, lean man who appears, like you, to be alone. The sun is so glaring you turn on your stomach and rest your head on your arm. You close your eyes and listen to the waves, the war cries, the transistor radio—and your own pulse throbbing in the ear pressed against your biceps. When you open your eyes you let them travel up and down your neighbor's body. His oiled flank has picked up orange dye from his beach towel. His profile glows in the bright, white light. His chest is almost hairless except for a fleur-de-lis of down around each nipple. His legs, however, are luxuriously furred and powerful. In a rush, that forbidden desire to touch his body comes over you.

Your neighbor has now turned on his side. The sun is so bright and strong you're not certain his eyes are trained on you. Now you can see how broad his shoulders are, and how narrow his hips, from which his muscular thighs project like arrows from a quiver, abristle with gold feathering. He *is* looking at you. He comes to your towel and asks you to oil his back.

He's staying at the hotel down the beach and after you've sunned for hours and jumped in the breakers and laughed and looked at each other and applied still more lotion to each other's bodies, he asks you up to his room for a lemonade. You feel you should tell him you're not . . . not what? Not attracted to him? Then how do you explain the embarrassing mound swelling your swim trunks? Sure, you'll come up for a drink.

He's very casual as you stroll through the lobby and ride up the elevator and you wonder whether you've been mistaken about him. After all, he *is* from out of town. He may have just stumbled by accident on the ''wrong'' end of the beach. You realize he's not guilty—a realization that makes you recognize that you are. No matter. He's a really good conversationalist, knows a lot about movies and music, has a great grin, a great . . . body.

Even in his room, once he's closed the door (at last!) he's still casual; never more so than when he steps naked out of his swimsuit and announces he's going to take a shower. ''Want to take one, too?'' he asks.

''Sure,'' you say with a nonchalant shrug and a throat dry enough to grow cactus in.

''Well then, come on.'' He leads the way.

You follow impatiently, reluctantly, gracefully, clumsily, happily, fearfully, as his brown body, with its band of white around the center, shimmers in and out of focus. Once you're both in the shower nothing could seem more natural than scrubbing his back and, as he slowly revolves, his chest. Some nagging little martinet in your brain keeps shaking his finger at you and gasping in shock, but you ignore the reprimands and move smoothly into his arms. His body is still hot from all the solar energy absorbed that day, glassy from the thundering water. Now his hair is wet and pressed against his skull, which turns out to be surprisingly delicate and finely shaped. He pulls you still closer, kisses you, and you're not certain whether you're drowning or in something very much like ecstasy. No man has ever kissed you like that before and it's odd to feel that bristly day's growth of

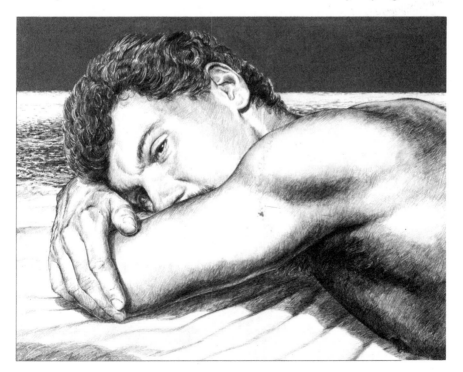

beard above the smooth lips. He backs off a second and says: "You're okay." All you can manage to do is nod, and hope he knows the nod means "Yes."

In bed you're so happy and so *relieved*—relieved of a cumbersome burden of yearning you've been shouldering too long—that you run your hands through your damp hair and just sigh.

"What's wrong?" he asks.

"Nothing," you tell him. "Everything's right. But I should tell you something. This is my first time with a guy."

"You could have fooled me," he says. "Do you want to stop?"

"In about two days."

He does think you should take a breather. Then you talk about your youth. You remember the years you jerked off to porno magazines and videotapes; lest you be ostracized by your peers for being a fag, you never showed too much attention to a friend in school. He has lots of interesting things to say, and his story is not too different from yours. That nagging little finger-shaker in your brain is less insistent. The talk is great, but what you really want is to get back into bed. At last you just say so and he says, "Sounds good to me."

He takes the lead in sex, and you don't explode, nor does the devil rise up out of the mattress to claim you. In fact, it feels good, but what feels best is this *freedom* to be next to another man. You can't believe you're finally free to touch him everywhere, to lie under him and on top of him, to kiss that sandpaper beard. Will it leave a beard burn? you wonder for a second of panic. Will people be able to *tell?* The panic gives way to a new surge of pleasure, the pleasure of inhaling another man, for surely that's what you're doing, that's what this freedom is, the freedom to breathe in the smell, the touch, the reality of an affectionate and sensitive man who seems to like you.

His jacket and slacks fit you, and after you're both dressed you go down to the dining room (no, the people can't tell, but, oddly, you wish they could). You feel a little formal and tired and relaxed after the sun and the sex—and the drama, taking place mainly in your head. Not much gets said over dinner, but looks are exchanged, and during coffee he squeezes your hand under the table. "I never thought," he says, "I'd be the one to bring someone out."

"To do what?" you ask.

"I just brought you out. Coming out. That means having your first gay experience."

The label sounds strange to you. You'd thought the word should be "freedom" or maybe "graduation." But of course that is what they—no, *we,* you suppose—yes, we gay guys call it: coming out.

The earliest urges toward homosexuality are usually exercised in adolescent fantasies. The homosexual aspect of some boys' fantasies may be disguised

—a boy may masturbate while imagining a man and a woman having sex, and may scarcely notice that most of his attention is focused on the man, zooming in for more close-ups of his anatomy than of hers.

Although some boys conjure up scenes of deep love and affection with members of the same sex, for most the fantasies are distinctly sexual. At puberty, boys think constantly about sex and generate powerful fantasies through masturbation. Society condemned masturbation for so long that even liberated people say little in its favor beyond assuring us there's nothing "wrong" about it. This latent puritanism has concealed what is very much *right* about the masturbatory fantasies through which adolescents explore which kinds of physical types and psychological characteristics are exciting. The jerk-off fantasy is a rehearsal, a preview of coming attractions, and it is a crucial learning experience (see *Masturbation and Fantasy*).

At some point the neophyte gay will have his first homosexual experience in the flesh. All the horniness held in check and vented only during masturbation will be released in a flood of desire. There is something very special about the initial sexual experiences. A few gays coming out confuse good sex with love. With maturity they learn that sex is not always a measure of love or intimacy.

After one or many experiences, someone coming out will have to say to himself, "I'm gay." To ever greater numbers of men entering gay life this statement comes naturally and easily. Others find self-acceptance harder to achieve, and the coming-out process takes longer. They may have sporadic sexual contacts, but they shrink from admitting their homosexuality even to themselves. Others think of themselves as gay, but do not let anyone else in on the secret (see *Homophobia*).

Of those who do come out publicly, some tell only one or two friends, others only members of their families; a few are open with everyone. Most often we disclose our homosexuality to parents, brothers and sisters, intimate friends, and, lately, employers, because we want no artificial barriers to stand between us and people important in our lives. If we come out to them with love, they are unlikely to remain distant for long, though some parents do demonstrate neurotic behavior when they learn of a son's homosexuality (see *Parents*). Even so, despite the risks, many sons feel the temporary stress is worth the bother if it eliminates the more pernicious stress of deception.

Perhaps the most harrowing part of telling others about our homosexuality is facing up to our own doubts and fears. If a gay man says, "I can't tell my parents because they believe homosexuals can never be happy," he may simply be attributing his own misgivings to them. It's easy to assign our own doubts to our parents, and it can be significantly counterproductive and downright wrong to do so. Many gays finally got up the nerve to come out to their folks only to hear, "We've known for years. We were wondering when you were going to find out you're gay."

So, coming out proceeds through stages, from fantasies to the first same-sex experience to acknowledging to yourself and then to others that you are gay, and finally to identifying with the gay community. How someone moves through these stages will differ from individual to individual and will be determined by several factors. How old you are and where you live will definitely make a difference. If you live in a small town, far from the big cities where homosexuality thrives openly, you may find little support in your efforts to come out. If you are a young man still living at home or if you are an older man whose whole mature life has been spent in the straight world, coming out can be painful. You'll need help from gay organizations and friends.

Homophobic religious training is another important determinant since condemnation by most religions remains very real. Ethnic and sociocultural factors can also influence coming out, both positively and negatively. (Read *Don't Be Afraid Anymore* by Troy Perry and *The Church and the Homosexual* by John McNeil.)

The current AIDS crisis is another impediment to young men coming out. Sexual excesses may reward a gay man with life-threatening illnesses, and who could blame him for turning away from contact out of fear and confusion? Men, young men in particular, search both for love and to satisfy a powerful libido, yet rightly fear their inexperience or foolishness will destroy them.

Gays just coming out have responded to HIV Disease with a number of sexual strategies. Some act as if they are omnipotent, invulnerable to human illnesses. This grandiosity is dangerous to themselves and to their sexual partners. At the opposite extreme are men who have taken vows of chastity, not because it's immoral, but in the belief that any sex is dangerous. Most gay men try to remain midway between these two extremes by meeting their sexual needs with responsibility.

HIV Disease has highlighted the responsibility we have as members of the gay community. Our first responsibility is to be informed about and to practice safe sex. The second is to encourage friends, lovers, and tricks to protect their own health. Finally, many gay men find that involvement in the community provides sustenance and meaning in their own lives. Consider joining an AIDS service organization and working with gay political groups that are fighting for our civil rights (see *Civil Rights; Gay Liberation*).

COMPUTER SEX

One doesn't have to be a computer expert to join an electronic bulletin board. There are at least five hundred such boards in America today. This modern technology can facilitate a wide variety of sexual contacts, and a few pieces of equipment are required. You need a computer (of any kind), a communications package (called software), and a modem, which connects the computer to the telephone line. So equipped, you can send and receive messages on any electronic bulletin board. As a rule, the "SysOp" (the systems operator, or guy who runs the board) will probably want to know a bit about you. You may also be required to pay a modest fee. This helps to keep out homophobic screwballs. The SysOp will ask you to choose a "handle," which is the name you'll use on the board. A person seldom uses his own; more likely he'll choose some fantasy name like "Hot Box" or "Randy Dandy." You can also change your handle when it no longer suits your needs.

All boards are composed of sub-boards. They include political discussions, social events, news, health, sexual fantasies, porno pictures—and member profiles. The profile board gives the "stats" on each member. Some boards show the stats as well, by presenting a picture of the member (*and his member*), front or back, hard or soft, naked or fully clothed. You give a description of yourself on the profile board. We suggest you don't lie if you want to meet people through the board. Be honest about your physical attributes. Express yourself creatively by letting everyone else on the board know what turns you on, what kind of men you're looking for, and what you'd like to do with them—and/or have them do to you. Once again, be honest, because boards are gossipy and you don't want to get a rep for being the kind of guy who misrepresents himself. One member of a gay board told so many lies about himself that other members refused to respond to his messages (or E-Mail, that is, electronic mail). So he "committed suicide," which is merely to say that he wrote a "suicide note" on the board so as to "kill off" his handle. Many letters of condolence were posted on the board afterward, and in all probability one of them was from the guy himself—using a new handle.

On the other hand, you may not want to meet people through the board. Your purpose may be only to have fun. Then, by all means, lie in your profile. Be directed only by your fantasies, and if Arnold Schwarzenegger is your idea of a man's man, then make yourself sound like the sexiest dude around.

Many boards have a "chat" function where two or more people can chat with each other on line. "Chatting" means typing away on the computer; what you type appears on the other man's screen. You don't actually talk to one another, and the anonymity provides a vast amount of fun for many people, especially those who are usually shy in social situations. If you chat, be friendly—dive in and "meet" new people. There's always an innate shyness at the beginning, and a certain degree of awkwardness when learning the keystroke commands to convey the message. In time it all gets sorted out, and shyness is transformed into bold sexual teasing. Beginners may want to do some "lurking" first. This means getting on a group chat line but not announcing yourself. It gives you a chance to see how others "talk" to each other. But they can tell that someone is lurking and you're bound to get invitations to join the discussion.

Some board members have sex together on the chat lines. Of course what's really happening is that they are jerking off while typing sexual comments to each other. Some members are quite inventive in making up really exciting scenes. This takes a bit of coordination since you're forced to juggle the lubricant and the tissues for the come while manipulating your dick and typing messages to your buddy. All the while you're trying to keep the lubricant and come from splashing your keyboard. If you're jerking off with someone this way, don't expect him to respond to your messages quickly. Like yourself, he needs a little time to stroke his dick and imagine what you look like and the sex you can have together. Some board members claim to get into "orgies" on the chat lines. This would seem to require a master of dexterity and imagination.

There are other sexual components to a board. Almost all have a picture section where you'll find soft-core and hard-core porno. These can be downloaded to your computer so you can look at them whenever you wish. If you're really attractive (or merely grandiose) you can have your picture posted for downloading. Some boards even separate the porno (it's called a GIF section) into sexual types, such as J.O., leather, fucking, and sucking.

About twenty-five gay boards in the United States have linked together into a network called GayCom. Private messages can be sent via GayCom from you to anyone who is a member of one of the other boards. This E-Mail is delivered overnight and it's far more reliable (often cheaper, too) than regular mail. Mail sent to you can be read on your computer screen and/or downloaded to your printer.

Computer boards use a whole new language to be learned, and it would all be quite solitary if it weren't for the bashes that most boards have: Members get together periodically just to have fun. Many gay men have developed love relationships after meeting other members at these bashes. And just about everyone finds new friends.

CONDOMS

It's not known how long condoms have been in existence. Some scholars claim to have found allusions to them in the works of Virgil and the Roman satirists. Condoms (and dildos) first appeared in England in 1660, supposedly brought over from Italy, and were in wide use by the eighteenth century, when sexually transmitted diseases had become rampant in Europe. By then they'd become so common that they were manufactured, openly sold, even advertised—as "implements of safety which secure the health"—in Paris and London. Mrs. Lewis held the London monopoly in the 1740s. By 1770 the monopoly passed to Mrs. Phillips, who became famous for her products. We find many references to condoms in the literature of the day: Samuel Johnson's biographer James Boswell casually writes in his journals of sexual encounters in which he was "unclad"

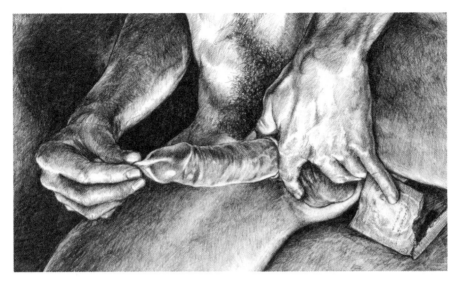

—i.e., not wearing a condom. The young author agonizes over whether he's contracted a venereal illness and will have to undergo a protracted and painful cure for "the clap" (see *Sexually Transmitted Diseases*).

Early condoms were expensive, if natural, products, usually made of lengths of sheep intestine sewn closed at one end and colorfully secured at the base with a red ribbon tied around the balls. Often ill-fitting and strong-smelling, they became increasingly expensive, rare, and difficult to obtain as rural areas shrank and sexual hypocrisy grew in strength during the Industrial Revolution. Late in the nineteenth century, rubber replaced animal gut as the condom material of choice, but these early products broke easily unless they were made so thick that most pleasurable sensations were completely dulled. The perfection of vulcanized rubber in the beginning of our century not only made possible the durable rubber tires that assured the ascendancy of the automobile in America, but also allowed for the cheaper, safer, thinner, and thus more pleasurable latex condoms so often found strewn around parking areas in various lovers' lanes.

By the Second World War, every kit handed out to the millions of men in the U.S. armed forces contained its share of "rubbers"—as latex condoms had come to be known—for protection against venereal disease. At the same time, the discovery of penicillin and antibiotics seemed to promise a future free of the worries that had afflicted our ancestors' sexual lives. Up to about 1970, young men still carried fold-up wallets indelibly deformed by the impression of a rolled-up Trojan, Sheik, or other brand of condom, but with a somewhat different intention: birth control. With the advent and instant popularity of the oral birth-control pill taken daily by women, condoms all but vanished from American life.

Condoms hadn't ever been in widespread use among homosexuals to begin with; when they entered gay sexual life at all, it was usually as a curiosity, a sex toy. Especially among those gay men who'd come out since the Stonewall rebellion of 1969 or who'd never had any heterosexual experience, condoms—if they were thought of or used at all—were considered kinky, sometimes a little daring. Now, however, with the spread of HIV Disease, condoms have become mandatory in our lives—truly a matter of life or death.

Also known as a rubber, a safe, a sheath, a comebag, a scumbag, a hat, a cap, a coat, or a capote, a condom is nothing more than a tube, usually made out of extremely thin latex rubber, with one end closed or slightly extended into a receptacle tip. Condoms are used during fucking, sucking, jerking off, and other sexual acts to receive and hold the come that shoots out of the cock opening (urethra). They provide an effective barrier against disease organisms.

Usually condoms are sold rolled up flat; they are about the size of a half-dollar coin and there is one condom per sealed package. Latex rubber, rather than "natural" or sheep-gut condoms, are the least permeable by bacteria and viruses and so the only safe type. Many condoms are sold prelubricated, some with nonoxynol-9 spermicide (sperm killer), for birth-control reasons and because the viruses believed responsible for HIV Disease are found in the living sperm cells that form part of the whitish fluid (semen) that comes out of the cock during an ejaculation. Only use a lubricant that contains nonoxynol-9.

When buying condoms you should read the information on the outside of the package and inspect the package to see that it's sealed tight. Most condom packages are dated. Check to see the date is current.

To put on a condom: Remove it from its package. Check the condom for any rips, tears, or perforations. Obviously this isn't always possible without breaking the mood established between you and your partner. Some men "wet" instantly, which is to say that they exude a lot of pre-come as soon as their cock gets hard. If you're one of these, skip the following few sentences. For those who are dry when hard, you might want to put a dab of lubricant on the inside of the condom. This makes it go on easier, and helps stimulate you during sex. Use *only* water-based lubricants such as K-Y or ForPlay. Don't use Crisco, baby oil, Vaseline, or any petroleum-based lubricants (see *Lubricants*). These work chemically against the latex and can make it degrade and tear. You can, however, use them for jerking off.

Holding the condom, place the head of your cock into the condom's opening and then slowly unroll it back along the cock shaft toward the body until it's on fully. It should fit snugly but not too tightly. It's important to hold the condom by its tip to prevent air from being trapped inside, as this could cause the condom to balloon out and rip. Condoms can catch painfully on genital hair, so go slowly.

When removing the condom, roll it over the head and off. Should you lose your hard-on when inside someone's ass, hold on to the base of the condom while pulling out. Some men use two condoms, one on top of the other. Those who use condoms while sucking prefer condoms without receptacle tips, as tips can get caught in teeth and tear.

Most condoms are made in one size. If your cock is too thick to fit into standard condoms or so narrow it flops around in them, you can find specially made condoms for you. Larger and wider sizes are known as max. Check in specialized sex-shops, which often go under the name of Pleasure Chest or Tool Chest. If you live in a rural area, look for condom ads in the pages of gay periodicals or straight sex magazines.

Be aware that condoms can break during long and rough bouts of ass-fucking. This is one area where it doesn't pay to be economical. Only use a condom once! Even if you didn't come in it, throw it out and put on another. It's a good idea to keep condoms handy. Those men who complain that putting on a condom "breaks the mood" obviously haven't tried having their sex partner put it on for them. If at the same time you lubricate each other and talk about your sexual fantasies, this can be a terrific turn-on.

If you've never used a condom before and are uncertain about using one, try it out alone, jerking off. Do this several times until you're comfortable with putting it on, and taking it off after you come.

Be aware that while there are controversies in current medical thinking, and while HIV Disease is now believed to be transmitted mostly through ass-fucking, safe sex guidelines recommend a condom even for sucking. This can be a problem because though many men complain about the lessened sensation while wearing a condom, few but rubber fetishists are interested in sucking a cock covered with one. Many get around this by not sucking or by not allowing their partner to come in their mouth. However, if you're someone who has a lot of pre-come, be safe and always use a condom while being sucked. And naturally it's always better to be safe than sorry. Don't, however, use a prelubricated condom. It tastes awful.

However experimental you want to get around this issue, *always* wear a condom for ass-fucking.

COUPLES

What is the origin of love? The Greek philosopher Plato answered this question in his *Symposium*. Plato has Aristophanes tell the following tale: In the beginning, there were three sexes: man, woman, and an androgynous man/woman. Each of the sexes was round, like a sphere, with a face and two arms and legs on either side. They could walk forward or backward, or tumble and roll on the ground. These three played and frolicked in the fields. But then they foolishly challenged the power of Zeus. For that, he punished them by splitting them in half, separating them, so there were two of each. What had been the double man (now two men), said Aristophanes, is the origin of gay male relationships; what had been the double woman (now two women) is the origin of lesbian relationships; and what had been the man/woman, now split into a man and a woman, is the origin of heterosexual relationships. Plato said this of the men:

> They who are a section of the male follow the male, and while they are young, being slices of the original man, they hang about men and embrace them, and they are themselves the best of boys and youth, because they have the most manly nature.

Aristophanes described the suffering of the three sexes after they were each split into two and separated. They felt as if their souls had been torn apart. Consequently, each spent all of its time searching for its other half, hoping to reunite. Each of the male halves was looking for his soul mate, and until he found it, he spent his days in sadness. Aristophanes said, *"The pursuit of the other half of one's self is called love."*

Today, we have the freedom to search for our soul mates, and, with luck, we may find our "other half." Love between two men gives them the strength to ignore the scorn of a heterosexual world, and immunizes them against a homophobic society. Gay love is a source of pride, courage, companionship, and security. Loving couples share more than their bodies. They share their souls.

There was a time when psychologists and psychiatrists claimed that gay men were incapable of real love, that their relationships were fated to break up because of emotional immaturity. There are probably still some professionals who maintain this biased belief despite all the evidence to the contrary. Long-lasting gay relationships are common in our society, especially since World War II. It's not unusual to meet white-haired men whose relationship has lasted fifty years or more. It's always interesting to hear how they explain the success and longevity of their relationships. One such man said, "You each have to forgive and forget a lot." Another said, "I keep his stomach full and his balls empty."

Some gay lovers would like their unions legally recognized. Though some steps have been taken in that direction, legal unions are not yet possible. Some municipalities now provide benefits for the spouses of their gay employees, as do a few private corporations (see *Civil Rights*). Perhaps the most significant advance in legitimating gay love relationships has taken place in the area of adoption. Thousands of children have been quietly adopted by gay men, and in many cities support groups for both fathers and children help sort out potential problems. A set of books for these children is now available from Alyson Press in Boston. (Read *Lesbian Moms, Gay Dads: Parenting a New Generation* by April Martin.)

Many problems in relationships are due to differences in personality type between the lovers. One, let's say, spends his energies on his home, furnishing and decorating it with panache. Out of a strong sense of attachment to his lover, he's building a nest, and he believes that love should last a lifetime. To him, intimacy with his lover is the highest achievement, and

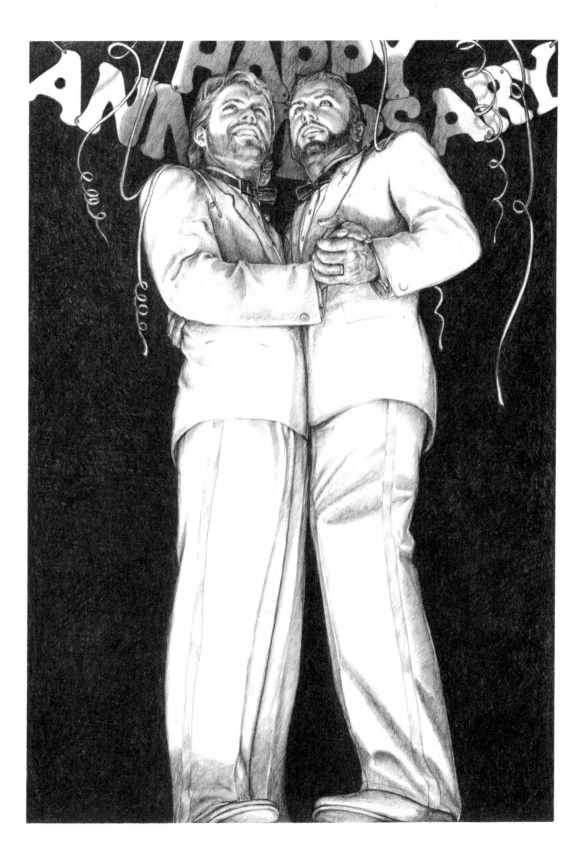

sex represents love. He agrees completely with the Greek lesbian poet, Sappho, who wrote about herself and her lover: "We came together like two drops of water."

A man with a different personality style, one who values autonomy and independence, is likely to be alarmed by the sentiment expressed in that quotation from Sappho. The idea of losing his individuality or merging his personality with another is repugnant to him. While he enjoys a comfortable home, his life is not focused on domesticity. And in sex, he likes excitement and novelty; he draws a distinction between lust and love.

The first personality described is characterized by what psychologists call *attachment;* the second, by what they call *autonomy.* The difference between these two styles is at the root of many conflicts between lovers. It's not that one is good or the other bad; it's the mismatch that causes problems. Two men who share the trait called attachment can make a happy couple, since their approaches to the relationship are similar. The same is true for two men who value autonomy in a relationship. Conflicts multiply when an attachment-motivated man sets up a relationship with someone autonomy-oriented. *Neither kind of man loves more than the other; they feel and express the love differently.* (A fuller explanation of these styles will be found in Silverstein's *Man to Man: Gay Couples in America.*)

No wonder sexual fidelity is the number one problem in gay relationships. Every couple faces the question of whether to maintain an exclusive sexual relationship (see *Fidelity and Monogamy*). Some lovers live together but have frequent sexual encounters outside the relationship. Sometimes these encounters are one-night stands; sometimes they involve steady partners. Many gay lovers who have been together for years and now seldom have sex with each other remain deeply committed, as in heterosexual marriages in the more sophisticated parts of Europe. These unions are known as *mariages blancs*, literally "white marriages."

The problem of sex outside the relationship also faces gay couples who are still having sex with each other. One partner, for instance, may be content to be faithful; his need for security may outweigh his desire for novelty. The other partner, however, may feel a strong desire for sexual adventure. In every case, a solution to the conflict can be found if the partners are willing to talk openly and honestly. Dishonesty is the chief enemy of good and enduring relationships: Partners who lie to each other are headed for disaster. Lying destroys mutual trust, and if two men do not trust each other, the relationship will not last.

Sex outside the relationship is particularly dangerous these days because of HIV Disease (see *Mixed-HIV Couples*). Each man has a responsibility not to bring HIV, or any other disease, into the relationship. Not surprisingly, many couples, regardless of their personality style, have agreed not to have outside sex, to eliminate the possibility of bringing disease into their home. On the other hand, couples who engage in outside affairs insist that each man follow safe sex guidelines.

There is another essential prerequisite for an ongoing, fruitful relationship: the realization that the relationship will change over time. When we find happiness with someone, we may feel that we have stumbled upon a magic formula that must be preserved. Accordingly, we resist change, unwilling to recognize that all living things, including relationships, must change or fall apart.

Gay couples also suffer from external pressures. In many places, bigotry still persists, and if it's linked to economic discrimination, the couple may break apart under the strain. The parents of one or both of the gay lovers may also undermine the relationship. Some parents may attack the relationship openly; more often they take a subtler tack: They pick a quarrel with the lover and force their son to take sides. Many parents, on the other hand, want their sons to be happy, and are supportive of their love relationships (see *Parents*).

Gay relationships commonly end because of personal conflicts. The primary psychological problem of our time is the fear of intimacy. Ironically, many couples break up because of their love for one another. One partner feels he is unworthy of love, and affection makes him frightened and suspicious ("He doesn't really love me, just his mistaken impression of me"). Another partner feels he is incapable of expressing love. Intimacy makes him feel guilty and inadequate ("He deserves someone better than me. I'm just a cold fish and I'm ruining his life").

More deeply, intimacy evokes feelings of vulnerability and loss of control in many men. Because they have been disappointed in their childhood relationships with their parents, or because they have been hurt in earlier love affairs, they may be alarmed when they sense a growing closeness to another man. This fear seldom expresses itself overtly. Often, it shows up in disguised forms, such as an inclination to pick absurd arguments or to suspect a partner of sexual infidelity, or even in a frantic urge to trick with strangers and thereby disrupt the love relationship. Sometimes the only way to deal with these fears is psychotherapy, perhaps together as a couple.

CRUISING

Looking for sex is called cruising and it can be done at any time and any place—over breakfast in a coffee shop, in a store while trying on shoes, at an exclusive reception, whether you're deliberately on the prowl or whether you're in the midst of errands and haphazardly find yourself in what seems to be an encounter. The most common time for cruising is at night and the usual places are those streets, parks, bars, and clubs where gay men congregate.

There's an art to cruising and its most important tools are timing and eyes. The eyes first: You're walking down the street and you pass a man going in the opposite direction. Your eyes lock but you keep on moving.

After a few paces, you glance back and see that he has stopped in front of a store window, but is looking directly at you. If he's not your type you'll probably register the compliment with a pleasant smile and leave. But if he does catch your fancy you may go through a little charade of examining the shop window nearest you. After a bit, the frequency and intensity of exchanged glances will increase, and one of you will stroll over to the other.

There are a few safe, stock opening lines, banal to the point of absurdity: "Have you got the time?" or "Got a light?" or "Where's Fourteenth Street?" After these preliminaries, introduce yourself, ask his name, and suggest you have a beverage together.

That, at least, was how cruising usually worked in the past. Today in big cities men often wear a "uniform" so distinctively gay (at least when they've set out to cruise) that there's no doubt about their orientation. Most people have become so open, casual, and fearless, the shop-window checking-out routine is skipped. You simply amble up to him and say, "Hi. Nice night, isn't it? You live around here?"

Once it's clear that one of you has an available space and both have the time and inclination, you're free to say "Let's go!" Many men, especially those with narrow sexual tastes, may ask, "What do you do?" when you first meet, and they don't mean for a living. Some answer the question immediately, while others feel that part of the fun of discovering a new person is finding out what he does in bed. The very lack of certainty adds spice to the encounter.

On the other hand, many men don't like to move right into sex without talking. It is not unusual to stop and chat over a cup of coffee. The conversation will not necessarily be sexual, but rather free-ranging and exploratory. You're getting to know something about each other—your background, job, and values, and other aspects of your life.

There are some practical advantages in chatting for a while. Suppose you're attracted to him, but you've heard disquieting stories about him. You might also feel there's something kinky, maybe even dangerous about him. A talk will give you a chance to size him up.

Should any of your fears be confirmed, or if after talking with him you lose interest DO NOT go home with him simply out of timidity or politeness. And NEVER HAVE SEX with anyone you're uncertain of, as this could lead to serious problems (see *Rape; Dangerous Sex*). Tradition has provided exit lines: "I had no idea it was getting so late; I've got to get home," or "I've got to meet a friend; give me your number and I'll call," or, more frankly, "I don't think it's going to work. Sorry." Exchanging phone numbers on the street isn't always a polite deception; sometimes one of you is actually in a rush and would genuinely like to get together later.

One recent and really very good (and even necessary) use of a conversation during cruising has to do with the AIDS crisis. You can use this talk to find out what and how much your potential sex partner knows about HIV Disease and safe sex. You can inquire about his own parameters of safe sex and whether they jibe with your own. For example, it might be that he won't have anal sex at all, but will have unprotected oral sex. Or he may be so frightened that he'll only indulge in voyeuristic masturbation from across the room.

Bar cruising is less matter-of-fact, more time-consuming, and often more frustrating. Everyone's reluctant to make the first move since he runs the risk of being rejected in full view of a room of other potential sex partners. As a result, the signals are as elaborate and subtle as the movements in Japanese Kabuki. He's interested in you, so he moves to your end of the bar, plants himself against the wall ten feet away, and grazes you with occasional glances. Your interest mounts and you move—not next to him, since that would make it awkward for him to look you over more closely— but to a position closer than before. At this point, if you stare you may scare him away; but if you ignore him too long, he may think you've lost interest. This languid mating dance progresses until one of you ventures a smile and the other returns it. The conventional opening lines in bars, such as "Come here often?" are often so familiar they're a joke. If the other guy has a sense of humor he'll laugh good-naturedly.

One real problem in getting anyone's attention even long enough to spout a cliché is the embarrassment of riches in bars. There are so many men to choose from, no one is willing to zero in on an individual who, after you've spent an hour chatting him up, may tell you he's got a lover. Then, too, Mr. Right may be the next man to come through the door. Another peril is socializing; some people are at the bar to see friends and have no interest in meeting anyone new. Finally, a few of those you see night after night propping up the bar want neither sex nor society; they're alcoholics, and all they want is another drink (see *Booze and Highs*; *Drugs*).

An extremely self-assured man can cut through the rigamarole of bar cruising, walk right up to someone and say, "You look interesting. Want to talk? Couldn't we do something better than stand here?" This approach can result in failure; the object of your interest may be startled or too conformist, and simply walk off without a word. Then again, he may light up with pleasure. Everyone secretly dreams of approaching a man in a bar and saying "Wanna fuck?" But few have pulled off that particular fantasy.

If someone rejects you after enticing you, don't worry about whether you said something wrong or ate too much garlic at dinner. He simply may not like your voice, or you may remind him of someone else, or he may not be wearing his contact lenses and so has made a mistake. More likely, you simply will not be his type (see *Types*). Or he may be a coquette. This annoying type haunts the bars and gets his kicks from turning people down; it's virtually a sexual thrill for him to say no, and after he's rejected three or four perfectly acceptable men he'll go home alone, fully satisfied (see *Rejection*).

A new kind of cruising involves the telephone. A man who can keep a public phone in view from his home can dial the booth when he sees someone attractive. If the man on the street picks up, the caller propositions him.

Car cruising is a national sport with several variants. In small towns and rural areas, rest stops in parks or along highways are often the main places for meeting other gay men. After the pickup the two may have sex in the woods, in a car, or at any other available spot. Another variant takes place when you're driving and notice someone attractive behind the wheel of a neighboring car. There are many ways to gain his attention.

Both types of cruising, however, hold inherent dangers. Arrest through entrapment at rest stops and public toilets is common in small towns, especially around election time. And those who prey upon gays often use these spots to meet unwary men. Be careful!

The term "compulsive cruising" applies when a man cruises every free moment; after he shows man one out the door, he returns to the street to look for another. There's less lust than longing in it. Maybe it's not about sex; maybe it's about loneliness. Maybe they're afraid of missing the Perfect Man. Perhaps they're caught in a self-defeating and downward-spiraling cycle: Gay sex makes them feel guilty, which makes them anxious, which makes them pound the pavements, which leads to more gay sex and more guilt. Often the compulsive cruiser *needs* love but *wants* sex. Since what he wants doesn't correspond with his need, he's restless and dissatisfied after sex and . . . he cruises. Such confusion and compulsion are agonizing and shouldn't be sneered at. But they needn't always be a sign of major trauma.

Many gay men may go through shorter periods of intense cruising in their lives: They're bored with their work or their social set; they're in a new town, in a new neighborhood, in a mood to meet new people and try different things. Cruising can be refreshing and put you onto a new track in life.

Taken in the right spirit and with the proper precautions, cruising can be rewarding and fun. You're meeting new people, forming new friendships, and expanding your sexual repertoire. More than one satisfied gay couple met through cruising.

DADDY-SON
FANTASIES

The "Daddy" scene has become rather popular these days. One finds porno videos and a magazine devoted to it. There's even a Daddy computer bulletin board in San Francisco (see *Computer Sex*). A couple of gay professionals have recently written about the importance of fathers in the sexual development of their sons. In 1981, Silverstein published *Man to Man: Gay Couples in America,* in which he documented the sexual interest some gay boys have in their fathers; some boys jerk off to fantasies of having sex with them. Occasionally, boys even attempt to seduce their fathers. In 1990 Richard Isay published *Being Homosexual: Gay*

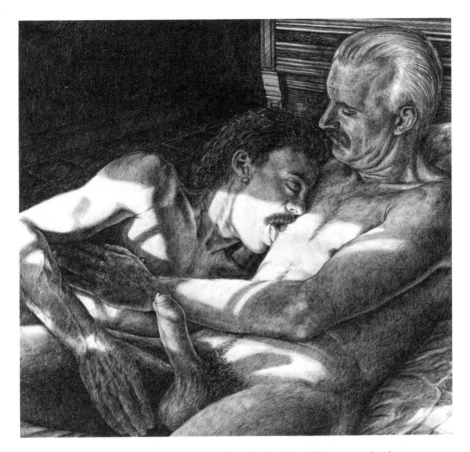

Men and Their Development, in which he further discusses the importance of the erotic attachment of gay sons to their fathers. (Read both of them.)

"Daddies" have certain physical characteristics. They have salt-and-pepper hair or thinning hair. They also have facial and chest hair. Their faces show maturity, and some "sons" prefer daddies with large hands. A Daddy doesn't have to be in good physical shape. The son isn't bound by age, but he does need to exude a boyish, even mischievous quality. While he may have facial hair, either he or his Daddy might prefer to shave his body hair (see *Shaving*).

The primary goal of Daddy-son scenes is taking care of the son, helping him to grow up within the context of a sexual scene. Occasionally the Daddy-son relationship continues outside of the bedroom as well.

The Daddy-son scenario is usually played out in the context of the son being either a "good boy" or a "bad boy." Naturally, bad boys are punished, often by ass-spanking over Daddy's knees (see *Spanking*). Sophisticates may go so far as to acquire and wear certain clothing: short pants for the "boy," a cardigan sweater and slippers for the "Dad." These accent the sexuality of the scene, as do belts and hairbrushes. Obviously clothing isn't required, as two naked men can play out the scene in bed perfectly well. Sons liked to get fucked by their Daddies and to follow Daddies' orders. Many of these scenarios end with the "boy" complimented for being "good"; the praise is, we suspect, the goal of Daddy-son scenes. For some gay men, perhaps those from unloving homes, the combination of being loved and fucked by Daddy is Nirvana.

The entire sexual scene is filled with talk between the two men, with the Daddy giving instructions to the son ("Show me how you can make Daddy proud"), and complimenting him for correct behavior. It's not unusual for the participants, particularly the son, to experience a great deal of emotion after coming. Cradled by his Daddy, the son may cry at the warmth and compassion he experiences, a warmth he probably never experienced with his biological father. You might want to subscribe to *Daddy: The Magazine,* Ganymede Press, Inc., PO Box 5325, Harrisburg, PA 17110-5325, for $18 a year.

DANGEROUS SEX

Danger lurks everywhere in life, including gay life, where a simple walk down the wrong street can turn you into a statistic of gay-bashing. While that may not be under your control, most other dangerous practices in gay life are. There are two main areas of potential danger: specific social behavior and specific sexual behavior. Both can be exciting—and can turn deadly.

There are some men who become aroused only when there's a danger they'll be arrested or hurt while having sex. Why such men should deliberately court disaster is undoubtedly as puzzling to them as it is to outsiders, and far more anguishing. Perhaps their first sexual experience occurred in a public place and the danger of discovery has, consequently, become eroticized.

The greatest danger—one that in some cases proves fatal—arises when a man is turned on only by encounters with straight teenage hoodlums or with psychopathic homosexuals. If you are excited only when you go into a notoriously dangerous public park at night, a place haunted by muggers and brutal teenage gangs, then you should analyze your sexual tastes before you are maimed or killed.

Another danger is the potential trick who feels compelled to tell you that "I'm really straight. I go for pussy." These disclaimers are a sure sign of a man who hates his homosexuality—and who may vent this anger on you in private.

The "foolhardiness" of men who put their lives in danger is not necessarily their characteristic way of dealing with the world. In business, with friends, and in all other nonsexual contexts they may be cautious and properly self-interested. But the sexual allure of danger—and especially the erotic fantasies touched off by the threat of danger—blind them and cripple their reality-testing abilities. For this reason they should seek psychotherapy.

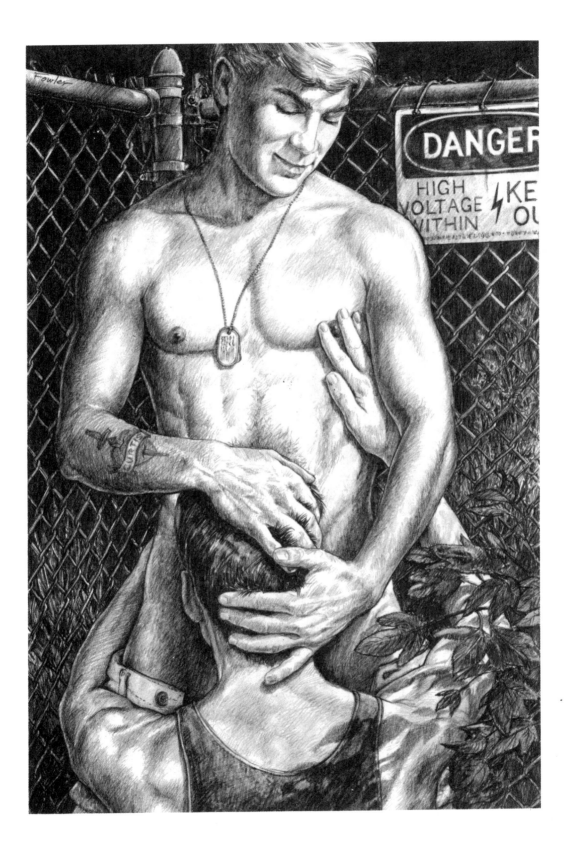

Some men also participate in forms of sexual behavior that are potentially dangerous. The most obvious example of dangerous sex today is engaging in unsafe sexual practices, such as not using condoms (see *Safe Sex*). Other unhealthy practices include not properly cleaning sex toys such as dildos and not making certain that skin piercing is performed under sterile conditions (see *Piercing*; *Sex Toys*).

A sexual behavior is definitely dangerous to one's safety if the practice is potentially infectious (see *Rimming; Scat*), if it damages the skin or organs of the body (see *Fisting*), or if it utilizes breakable objects, such as glass rods inserted into the urethra. Sometimes these practices can be embarrassing as well as dangerous. One unfortunate soldier was found with his dick snared up the tube of his bayonet sheath, while another man was rescued when his dick was stuck up the faucet in his bathtub. Social scientists know very little about the origin of these exotic ways to satisfy the libido, which are called *paraphilias*. The term means "faulty loves." They all have this in common: Behavior thought of as either disgusting, distasteful, or physically painful by society at large becomes charged with sexual excitement.

One paraphilia is as dangerous as getting beaten up in the park. It's called *autoerotic asphyxiation*. It's an unusual form of masturbation that sometimes results in death. In one technique the masturbator literally hangs himself while jerking off. The masturbator progressively closes off his windpipe, aiming toward something known as the blue light, a mental-physical state in which mental awareness is supposedly increasingly limited and physical concentration is supposedly intensified, leading to an intense orgasm. The obvious problem is that the masturbator may not be able to release the noose after he comes, and so falls first into unconsciousness, then death.

Professionals have no idea how such an idiosyncratic form of challenging the Reaper originated, nor do they know how to change it. But it's evident that the alleged delights have made this paraphilia popular, especially among suburban and rural adolescents, who often perform it while stoned on grass or alcohol and wearing headphones that are blaring out heavy-metal rock music. Deaths do occur, and the nude or semi-clad bodies of brothers or sons are found by startled families. (Read *Lovemaps* and *Vandalized Lovemaps,* both by John Money.)

Good judgment is the best rule for avoiding danger. This includes making choices about tricks, lovers, and sexual practices. There are unquestionably some men who function effectively in the world of paraphilias, giving and receiving sexual pleasure without danger. There are others, however, whose safety is in question. We hope that they will seek out friends or therapists with whom they can talk, and that ultimately they will either give up the behavior or learn to appreciate the excitement of sex without danger to their lives.

DEPRESSION

Depression is the feeling that no one in the whole world understands or cares for you. It occurs when you have no one around to praise you, or when you are unable to accept or to believe in the praise you receive. Often it follows a sudden and radical loss of status (either real or perceived)—conflict with one's family, say, or the loss of a job—and it is a particularly common consequence of hopeless love affairs or the death of a loved one.

Depression is different from sadness, what some people call "feeling blue." Sadness is always a response to a real tragedy, and the feeling of loss is appropriate. People who are sad grieve for the loss of a friend, a family member, or even a job, but then, after grieving, move on (see *Letting Go*). It is when a person cannot let go of the sadness that he transforms himself from feeling blue to being depressed, or moves, as some depressed people say, into blackness.

Psychoanalysts commonly say that depression is a repressed form of anger, a deflection of hostility away from its external object onto oneself. Whether this theory is accurate or not, venting of anger is often the best way to overcome depression, since expressing anger reverses and banishes the sense of powerlessness. When you assert yourself, you once again feel effective and worthwhile.

This psychoanalytic theory is probably too unidimensional to explain the pervasiveness of depression in gay men. Clearly one cause of depression is the effect of homophobia, and we call the result *learned depression*. Gay men are often taught from childhood that they disappointed their parents by not being butch or conforming enough; are taught by their faith that they are sinners; are taught by the law that they are lawbreakers. One readily understands why many gay men have grown up feeling depressed about their homosexuality. A young man feeling rejected and unloved by parents, siblings, peers, and the community at large could hardly feel otherwise (see *Homophobia*).

There are two other causes of depression, though both are still speculative at this time. Some men may have a biological predisposition to depression, possibly inherited from the father. Other men adopt a depressed attitude from a parent by a process called *identification*. This means that the young boy internalizes his mother's or father's own low self-esteem and feelings of inadequacy.

Biological depression can be physically as well as psychologically painful, and medication is almost always helpful. Any form of depression can be so damaging to one's self-esteem that suicidal ideas become common, and in some cases are acted upon.

The depressed gay man often turns to sex for comfort and relief, but in sex he does not find the solace he is seeking. What a depressed person really needs is affection and closeness. As a sexual partner, someone who is depressed isn't much good. He's so compliant that he's inactive during sex, and this excessive passivity just isn't very sexy. The depressed person sends out signals that baffle his partner. Disappointed after sex because he has not received the simple affection and affirmation he needs, a depressed person emits signs of his disappointment that confuse and wound his partner.

Yet touching is precisely what the depressed person needs most, though the form the contact takes may be holding instead of fucking, stroking instead of sucking. If you're depressed, ask someone to hold you. The person you ask will probably be a friend or lover, but, surprisingly, even strangers can be moved and flattered when requested. Animal comfort, however, is not enough. If you are depressed you need to be with people who like you, who value your opinions, who see things from your point of view. Being a loner may seem a romantic pose, but when you're depressed you should abandon it and be with friends.

Many gay men become depressed when they are rejected sexually. If someone is already depressed, he can interpret the least sign of indifference as a rejection. A depressed or insecure man trying to make out in a bar, say, ensures his failure by going, with an unerring instinct for defeat, straight to the coldest stranger in the room. By contrast, someone in a buoyant frame of mind is relaxed, a bit choosy, and ready to admit that his appeal is not universal. He knows that this guy may go only for diminutive blonds, that one for overweight lawyers, and that one over there only for money (see *Types*). But a depressed person is frantic and quite forgets the bewildering range of human sexual preferences. He never stops to say to himself, ''But I may not be this fellow's type,'' or ''That guy may not want to go home with anyone if he has to get up early tomorrow for work.'' Rather, he makes nervous overtures in every direction and translates the first no into a total dismissal of his entire value as a human being.

A few gay men are depressed after sex, especially after sex with a trick. Sometimes the partner is a warm, affectionate person, but this very warmth can be threatening to a person afraid of intimacy. He gets rid of the trick as quickly as possible—and then vaguely senses he has lost yet another opportunity to connect with another person and develop a rewarding relationship.

There are a number of good treatments for depression. New medications are very helpful, especially in combination with psychotherapy.

DIRTY TALK

Sex is not a simple agitation of the loins, a few squeals, a tussle, an ejaculation, and then the slow resumption of grazing on the meadow. All human actions beyond a few reflexes have been shaped by learning and as a result, the same erotic combinations can be interpreted in hundreds of different ways, according to the value the imagination attaches to them.

That's where dirty talk comes in. Because we are creatures whose lives are caught in a net of words, naming the very act we are performing heightens our excitement. Dirty talk creates the act as it describes it, for talk is one of the most potent means for changing straightforward sex into a defilement, or a childhood prank, or an obscenity or a religious rite.

Dirty talk, whether it is occasional bursts of four-letter words or the unwinding of an elaborate fantasy, whether it's all one-sided or a collaboration, enhances communication, for through it you can instruct your partner in your sexual needs. For many men, going to bed with a guy who has a really filthy mouth is the ultimate turn-on.

If you have trouble getting started, try this: Start off by describing what you're doing sexually to your partner. Then, as you go along, put more feeling into the words. Pretty soon you'll notice that your partner is squealing in delight—and throwing a few words your way.

DOGGY STYLE

This is the classic gay fucking position, the reality behind those old jokes about never turning your back on a Greek and behind facetiously saying "I kept dropping my soap in the shower—hoping something would happen." In doggy style, you drop to your hands and knees, and he enters you from behind. For some men it's the preferred position: After all, it's the one doctors have you assume for a rectal exami-

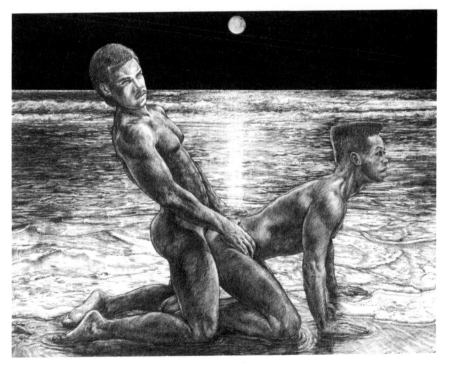

nation, because it affords the easiest entry. For the man doing the fucking, doggy style enables him to make pelvic thrusts at the fastest possible rate; for pure speed it can't be beat. And due to the angle, for many men it is the best position for fucking deeply and over the longest period of time.

It's also a very sexy position. The man on top has a full view of the buns he's penetrating and he can watch his own cock slide in and out of his partner's asshole. He can let his gaze wander slowly up his partner's back and stop at the tensed shoulders and straining triceps, or he can lean over and wrap his arms around his partner's waist or chest and nibble at his exposed nape or ear. The guy getting fucked is possibly more conscious of his own body in the doggy position than when he is lying on his back (see *Face-to-Face*) or on his stomach (see *Bottoms Up*). The fuckee is also more active in this position. He can push back onto his partner's cock; he can rest his weight on one forearm, freeing his other hand for masturbating himself. Or he can easily drop down from all fours to stretch out on his belly, and from there roll his partner and himself onto their sides (see *Side by Side*). Or while still up on all fours, he can raise his upper body until both he and his partner are kneeling, hips, torsos, and heads vertical. This is a great position from which to turn and kiss.

Kissing, however, is a casualty of fucking doggy style: Unless the bottom has a rubber neck or the top is extraordinarily tall, a full mouth-to-mouth kiss is virtually impossible (see *Kissing*).

DOMESTIC VIOLENCE

*L**over battery** is a form of domestic violence that is no different in its etiology and effects than wife-beating and child-beating. Battery usually begins with an occasional slap or "loving" punch, which is often explained away, or "not meant." Apologies and even lovemaking follow. As the batterer finds himself getting away with it, his lover finds the abuse increasing week after week, with the alleged reason for the slap or kick or punch becoming more trivial.

As the battering continues, the lover finds himself fearing punishment for any behavior not approved by his battering partner. He finds himself doing virtually everything to please his lover and to avoid being hit. He also finds himself in the odd and humiliating position of making alibis for, lying about, and even excusing his lover's behavior to others who notice his bruises. He may even come to blame himself for his stupidity, his ineptitude, which is, after all, why his lover tells him he's being hit: a loving chastisement geared toward making him a better person, a more appropriate lover.

At last, the battered lover finds himself living in fear for life and limb, yet unable to tear himself away from the man who passionately kisses him one minute and severely punishes him the next.

What is really going on in such a relationship? Doubtless, homophobia in some form; probably, self-hatred passed on as hostility toward the partner. For the victim it may be the secret fear of never being worthy of love that transforms him into a punching bag for someone else's fears and anxieties. (Read *Growing Up Gay in a Dysfunctional Family* by Rik Isensee.)

Who becomes a battered lover? Anyone. You can be intelligent, cultured, rich, brilliant, or famous. Who becomes a battering lover? Here the list is a bit shorter. The potential exists in many gay men, especially homophobic ones and those who harbor resentment and hostility, blaming others for their own deficiencies. Alcohol and drugs are often contributors; the mix of alcohol and hostility can end in physical abuse.

Does your lover have a short fuse? Does he lose his temper easily? Does he hit things and pets? Does he break and throw objects around the house or apartment? Does he verbally abuse others? Has he become overly jealous and possessive? If that picture fits your lover and over a period of time he's begun hitting you often (even if he cries afterward and begs your forgiveness), it's time to get the hell out of that relationship, fast!

How do you do it? Get a trusted friend to help. You might also call a domestic-violence hot line. Don't tell your lover, since he'll only cry and apologize once again—and beat you all the more the next time he's angry.

Arrange with your trusted helper to get away from your lover with as many of your belongings as possible. If you have to, get out with nothing but the clothes on your back. Do not go where he will expect you to go. Find a new place to stay. Make certain your battering lover doesn't know where you are and can't find out.

Stay away from him. Accept no phone calls or letters. If you must see him to settle business matters, see him *only in a public place* and with another person at your side. *Never see him alone!*

It's more than probable that this guy will go on to find someone else to abuse, and you may find yourself wondering whether or not to warn the new lover. The new lover will no more be able to accept your warnings than you could accept the warnings of your friends. Last, get into psychotherapy and learn why you chose an abusive lover, so that you won't repeat it.

DRUGS

Gays began using recreational drugs during the late sixties, when they became widely available through the counterculture. The real innovation in drug use, however, occurred during the seventies, the disco era: a specific kind of carefully graduated drug use called drug contouring or designer drugs. In the last few years younger gays have returned to this kind of drug use. A recent article in the *New York Times* showed cocaine use way down and LSD use way up. Reports of those users who end up in emergency wards confirm this pattern has revived strongly.

"Contouring" meant that you recognized the specific properties and effects of each drug and put them into your body in a particular order and at specific intervals, thereby enhancing your evening out in the club, a sexual encounter, or your afternoon in the park.

Thus, in those days, you might have decided to use LSD-25 for the night. Since LSD is a powerful, long-lasting (eight to ten hours) drug with several physical and mental side effects, you would probably be able to party all night with undiminished energy. On the other hand, you'd plan to sleep most of the following day, drink lots of fruit juices (while on the drug and afterward), and eat well to replenish the vitamins and minerals leached out of your body during the trip. Because the initial effect of the LSD was quite intense, you might have prepared the way, toning it down beforehand with drugs like marijuana and wine; these might also have been used during the course of the LSD trip if it became too rocky. At the end of the evening, in order to come down and to control some of the nervous energy still available, you might have taken a stronger depressant. Hypnotics like Quāā-ludes and Mandrax became especially popular because they allowed you to be responsive to rhythmical activity such as dancing and sex—always a nice way to end a trip. Unfortunately, taken by themselves rather than as part of the design, and taken in quantity, Quāāludes and Mandrax could also become physically addictive.

A smaller "arc" of designer drugs could be put together for shorter and less intense periods of time. Some people never used the stronger hallucinogens—also called party drugs—like LSD, MDA, or Ecstasy, but concentrated on grass or hashish. For them, contouring meant using a light amount of an "up"—a few snorts of cocaine, say—to help them to a more active state than that induced by grass. Or they might have sniffed poppers—amyl or butyl nitrate—during dancing or sex for a peak in their high. A few became dependent upon poppers.

A decade ago, gay resorts like the Fire Island Pines, Key West, and Provincetown were used by underground drug entrepreneurs to test out new recreational drugs. The dealers still sometimes go to these places and offer free new drugs to people in the party crowd. Ecstasy, MDA, rubber, Special K, angel dust, and PCP all made their debuts this way, and were judged by connoisseurs the way a new vintage is judged by expert wine tasters. Some made the grade and are widely used today, while others were found to have unpleasant side effects—angel dust caused paranoia and extreme disorientation, for example—and faded into oblivion.

As survivors of the disco era discovered, whenever you're using recreational drugs it's best to begin with a large dose of common sense. All physically addictive drugs should be avoided. That includes derivatives such as heroin, cocaine, and crack. Also addictive are the amphetamines, such as methedrine, crystal, and all other ups. The downs—barbiturates—include Tuinal, Seconal, Nembutal, and almost all other sleeping pills and are also addictive. Downs can be life-threatening; the withdrawal process for those addicted to them must be medically supervised, or death may result. These addictions almost always end in disaster for the addict and his loved ones. Some drugs are more obviously destructive—crack, for example, or heroin. Others seem more innocent but in fact are far more insidious.

Cocaine often becomes the drug of choice for gay men with low self-esteem, poor self-image, and self-hating homosexuals. Taken often enough, cocaine eliminates inhibitions. The user sees himself as a social success, a brilliant talker, or an expressive genius. And in fact, at the beginning, the drug's release of long-held inhibitions may actually make those using it seem much more personable and outgoing. But the cocaine user soon discovers he must continue using larger amounts of the drug to sustain that fragile new sense of self-worth: a scenario for addiction.

Before you take drugs, determine which of these three categories you fit into: the user, the abuser, or the addict (see *Booze and Highs*).

Drug strengths can vary widely. Always make sure that someone not using the drug knows you're on it, that he can be immediately contacted, and that he can be relied upon to help you if you have a severe reaction to the drug. This may mean having a designated driver. But some stronger hallucinogenic drugs require "guides" to help the first-time (or even tenth-time) user of the drug through the varied stages of the drug trip, which could be frightening. This is *very* important.

Don't take drugs from strangers. Ever.

Don't insist that someone in your group, someone you're seeing, or someone you've just met also take the drug you're on. Despite how great you may feel and how much you may want them to share your experience, don't!

Finally, recognize that the use of alcohol or drugs is the leading reason why gay men have unsafe sex (see *Safe Sex*).

EARLY ABUSE

"The Child is father of the Man," said William Wordsworth, and we couldn't agree more that childhood experiences lay important foundations for adult sexuality. Unfortunately, some of us come from dysfunctional families where we experienced physical, verbal, or sexual abuse.

There are many reasons why children are abused. Emotionally disturbed and alcohol- and drug-dependent parents often terrorize their children simply because they are the handiest objects. Some parents sexually exploit their children (see *Rape*). More subtle damage occurs when children are brought up in families where parents and children hide all feelings from one another, performing only the mechanics of family life as though they were actors on a stage. No wonder children born into these families grow up with a well-honed mistrust, and in adulthood, become overcontrolled in love and sex.

A few gay men blame their homosexuality on an abusive father, but this notion is merely internalized homophobia. More often one finds gay men feeling guilty about their erotic life. Oddly, some men counter these feelings by an obsessive sexual feast composed of nameless men and blank faces, night after unsatisfying night. One such man said that for him it was "affection at any price." A few men solve their conflicting sexual feelings through celibacy, others by carefully controlling what sexual acts they'll perform, usually a limited lot. But all these men suffer one limitation in common: They cannot feel intimate with another man. Control becomes their substitute for vulnerability, even when they're in the arms of a loving, caring partner.

The problem is how to get them to separate early abuse from adult sexuality. A number of obstacles intervene. A man may choose lovers every bit as abusive as his father (see *Domestic Violence*). Friends sadly marvel at the phenomenon, seeing their best counsel ignored while their friend runs from one abusive lover to the next.

But most men choose lovers more wisely. Even so, their sex life may be strained and rigid. Ellen Ratner, author of *The Other Side of the Family: A Book for Recovering from Abuse*, tells us: "The instrument of pleasure (the body), is also that which holds the pain." She means that the formerly abused man can't let go sexually, because by doing so, he'll reexperience the painful abuse of childhood. It is as if his memory were contained within his muscles, rather than in his brain. Memories of being abused may return during sex with a lover, perhaps as a quick flashback or in reaction to smelling an article of clothing. Psychologists call these reminders *triggers*.

If you were abused in childhood, you should consider looking into psychotherapy and joining a support group. If your memory of that abuse is interfering with your sex life with your lover, ask him to be part of the therapeutic process. Otherwise, he'll have trouble understanding how you can be ashamed and uptight at the same time that you're aroused. You may understand that your discomfort isn't your partner's fault, but he may not.

In the meantime there are things you and your partner can do to help bring more complete trust into the relationship. You might try "Simon Says." You, the abused partner, say: "Touch my _____." Depending on how it feels to you, continue or discontinue the touching. Do it clothed or naked, as you wish. Another technique is to outline a body on a piece of cardboard and to identify the body parts that feel good to you when touched, and those that don't. Color them differently, and change colors as you feel more comfortable sexually. Try taking your partner's hand and moving it along your body and telling him what kind of touch and which places on your body feel safe. Finally, develop trust by trying a "blind walk." Your lover blindfolds you, and then leads you by the hand around your apartment, stopping from place to place to let you feel objects and guess what they are. If you live in a rural area, go outside and touch flowers or leaves. Then reverse roles by leading him in a blind walk.

EFFEMINACY

No one is sure whether male children are born with or learn effeminate behavior. We suspect that some traditionally feminine characteristics are biologically determined in some gay men. Their feminine traits and interests are as natural to them as an interest in baseball is to the stereotypical boy. In school, these boys are taunted constantly and mocked as "sissies." They get rejected by peers, teachers, and in some cases, their own parents. Repeatedly told to "butch up" their act, they come to believe that there isn't anything right about them. This effeminacy is part of their character and it remains throughout life.

In a different set of boys, learning seems to be the primary ingredient. Here, young men coming out who never expressed effeminate behavior in childhood do so in adolescence. Is this because the necessity of acting "like a man" is no longer operative and they can act as girlish as they like? Perhaps it's a way to take revenge on parents. It's rare that such behavior lasts very long; usually it disappears as they become more at ease with their sexuality. Some of it is just camping.

Some men are strongly attracted to effeminate gays. Perhaps they find them less of a threat to their egos than a masculine-looking gay man, or perhaps they identify with stereotypical ideas of marriage.

Effeminacy is by no means limited to gay men. One will also find straight effeminate boys who are taken for gay and discriminated against as fully as are gay boys. From grade school right through adult life, it is the effeminate child who is perceived as different from other males and who is bullied and beaten up. Regrettably, even adult gay men may discriminate against an effeminate man.

There are gay men who refuse to associate with others who have feminine traits. "He's too femme," they say, to rationalize their ostracism. This attitude is an expression of homophobia based upon the traditional notion of a strong and impermeable barrier between male and female behavior (see *Homophobia*). If you find yourself uncomfortable in the company of men with feminine traits, don't blame it on them. Instead, ask yourself why you're afraid.

FACE-TO-FACE

Facing your partner while you fuck is the position preferred over all others by most gay men. You can look at each other, you can kiss, you can read each other's faces for cues or just for the visible signs of pleasure given and received. For some men, face-to-face is also the position that enables the deepest possible penetration.

Some men find the penetration *too* deep (see *First Time*). Others dislike getting fucked in this position because they feel passive or feminized, while

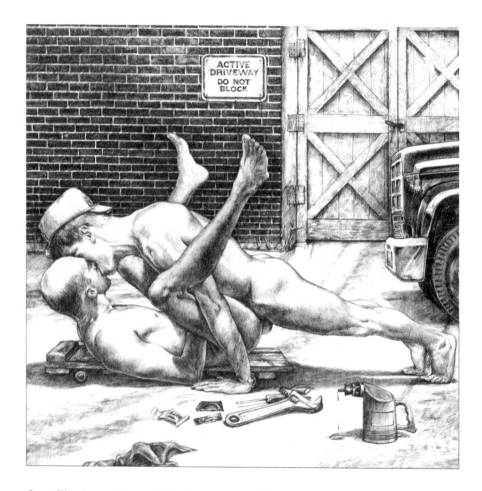

for still others, the passivity is a turn-on. Some object to face-to-face fucking on more practical grounds: Their legs become cramped. If sex goes on for a long time, the man on the bottom may get tired of having his legs hooked over his partner's shoulders and his knees pressed to his own chest.

When you are both fully aroused and at ease, stimulate and relax your partner's anus with your finger, and insert a lubricant into his asshole. Then, after you've place a condom on your cock, he's ready to be fucked (see *Condoms*). Formerly, many men liked to rim the asshole, since tongue stimulation is highly pleasurable to both parties, and also because the saliva serves as a good lubricant. Unfortunately it also increases the chance of infection (see *Rimming, Sit on My Face*). Kneel between his legs, lift his ankles, and place them on your shoulders. He may prefer his right foot hooked over your shoulder, his left foot below, wrapping around your back; this position gives more flexibility, and it places his asshole at a slightly different angle in relation to your cock, which may facilitate entry.

While fucking face-to-face can be the most exciting of sexual acts between men, getting inside in this position is where most problems occur.

Guys of different sizes, shapes, and weights can often encounter real problems. But with a little patience, and a will to succeed, no problem is insuperable. You may be really raring to go, but calm down a bit and be tolerant of your partner's comfort: You'll both enjoy it better.

Entry should be slow and gentle, allowing his sphincter muscles to relax to accommodate your cock. Once you are all the way in and he feels comfortable, you can bend over and kiss or tongue any part of his upper body. And if you both are comfy, you're also ready to try hard-thrust fucking. Some guys really like this and shout and slap each other's buttocks to increase the excitement as they get closer to climax (see *Spanking*).

If you're both agile and your bodies fit together in a particular way, it may also be possible to fuck and suck him at the same time. Sit back on your heels, simultaneously pulling your partner up onto your lap; he should wrap his legs around your waist. The lower his legs, the more direct the pressure against his prostate gland and the more pressure (and thus pleasure) he feels. He should not try to sit up to fold his arms around your neck (that's another position, which has its own merits), but continue to lie on his back on the mattress, while his pelvic area is propped up on your thighs.

If you now bend your head down to his crotch, you should be able to suck his cock. You may have to angle his cock down, or you may have to use your other hand to form an extension to your mouth (see *Blow Job*). You won't be able to deep-thrust but you can get some movement. Try this: As you pull out your cock, go down on him. As you push back in, lift your mouth away. Or you can jerk him off as you fuck.

For deep fucking, bend him back until his knees nearly touch his shoulders. His weight will rest on his spine and neck, and his ass will stick straight up. Go up on your toes and fingertips, as though doing push-ups. Grasp his ankles and open his legs wide without forcing. You may have to balance yourself by shifting your weight from your toes to your knees.

Another position: Stand or half-crouch on the floor beside the bed (you may want to elevate your partner slightly by placing a pillow under him). His back will rest on the mattress, but his legs will be straight up against your chest. To avoid losing your balance, lean over and steady yourself against the wall. An alternative is for you to grab his ankles and open his legs as wide as possible, relying on the resistance of his body to keep you from falling over on top of him. If you're strong, you can even lift your partner off the bed and carry him around while still inside him.

If you are the one getting fucked, and your partner is masturbating you and you sense you're about to come, gently move his hand away, and jerk yourself off. This will help you achieve an orgasm simultaneous with his. But if your legs or back begin to ache, don't grin and bear it; tell your partner you want to rest or try something else.

Face-to-face admits variability of sexual and emotional expression, and partners can move from gentle, cherishing tenderness to athletic roughness.

No matter what your scene, being fucked takes getting used to. If you have lower-back problems you may want to avoid it altogether or warm up to it slowly. Remember, tell your partner what feels good, adjust your position, and find the most pleasurable angle.

FETISH

In sexual terms, a fetish can be anything not manifestly sexual that has been invested with erotic appeal. For instance, a man whose first physical contact with other men occurred in sports may make a fetish out of football helmets or jockstraps, while a man who has cast long looks from windows at telephone repairmen or construction workers may eroticize hard hats, or utility belts festooned with tools. Leather—its look, smell, and feel—is a familiar fetish, and for some men one whiff of cowhide can induce an erection. (Read *The Leatherman's Handbook II* by Larry Townsend.) A certain brand of underwear (or, better yet, used underwear or jockstraps), thick white athletic socks, boots or workshoes, feet, belts, cow-

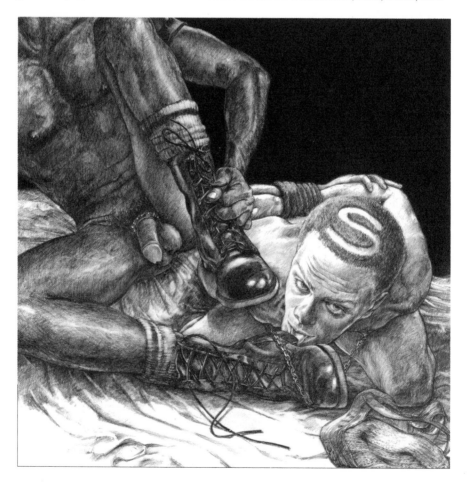

boy shirts, the smell of French cigarettes—any of these can pick up erotic associations.

Most of these are the trappings of maleness in its many varieties, but some gay men have made fetishes of women's panties or lace slips or dresses, and nothing seems more desirable to them than their own bodies, or other men's, in drag. And in fact, since gay liberation it seems as though the body itself, worked out in a gym to be well muscled and perfectly tanned, has become fetishized. Some men have been known to fall in love because of a specific configuration of stomach muscles (the "washboard"); others fall for men whose biceps, deltoids, legs ("thunder thighs"), or large buttocks ("bubble butts") are particularly well developed.

Most of these fetishes are really no more than specific preferences. When you are in the presence of an attractive man but lack the preferred object, you'll have sex anyway and be satisfied.

It is only when a specific fetish must *always* be present, and when it becomes more important than the presence of a sexual partner, that it becomes psychologically limiting. If, for example, you like to masturbate while sniffing a jock, and the jock becomes preferred over another person, then the fetish is taking over your sexuality. The likely aftereffect is loneliness. Should that happen, therapy is in order, with the goal of integrating the fetish into sexual contact with other men.

Some excellent twentieth-century fiction has been written about fetishes: the Japanese novelist Junichiro Tanizaki has explored foot fetishes, tattooing, and so on in *Seven Japanese Tales* and *The Secret History of the Lord of Musashi.*

FIDELITY AND MONOGAMY

They are not necessarily the same. Fidelity between lovers excludes the possibility of having sex with a third person; monogamy means that two people have declared themselves lovers—an intimate emotional and sexual relationship. The latter arrangement can include sexual adventures outside the relationship. Not surprisingly, some couples, especially during the health crisis, insist the terms are synonymous: no sex outside the relationship.

Arguments about fidelity are the commonest reason that couples break up (see *Couples*). Gay men are subject to the same emotional ideology as straights, which means they often maintain mistaken notions of possession of the partner—each owns the other's body, just as in some forms of marriage the husband has direct rights of ownership over the wife (see *Jealousy, Envy, and Possessiveness*). Movies, books, and poems all bolster the idea that love is possession, and this confusion between them often underlies disputes about infidelity.

Sort out your feelings if you suspect your lover of infidelity. Jealousy can be the product not only of possessiveness but also of a lack of confidence in yourself. The fear is that if your lover has sex with others he may find someone more exciting than you. Jealousy may be a mask for envy; perhaps you believe he is more attractive than you and is having more success.

Lovers need to be explicit in devising rules to suit each other's needs and vulnerabilities. That requires honest (not cruel), possibly lengthy (not tedious) conversations; in a love relationship there are responsibilities as well as opportunities.

It's always complicated for lovers to set up rules about having outside sex, since each of them fears abandonment. That's all the more reason why they should agree on the parameters. Sometimes a settled couple will set up a rule that if they go out together for an evening they will always return home with each other. If one meets someone he likes, he may take that person's phone number and make arrangements for getting together, but he may not desert his lover during their night out. Some partners have a rule that they will have sex with outsiders only in threesomes that include the other lover; others, that they will trick out only when one of them is out of town. Still others stipulate that a trick cannot be brought home. Such rules can and should change as the relationship evolves, as it is bound to do, and as the lovers discover and come to accommodate each other's needs.

One should also note that there have always been gay couples who have insisted on both fidelity and monogamy, adhering to the belief that gay lover relationships, like heterosexual marriages, exclude outside sex. Though many find it hard to believe, there are numerous examples of sexual fidelity in gay relationships.

To a different set of men, tricking out represents health dangers. They fear the HIV virus may be introduced into their relationship by a third party and they've sworn off tricking "for the duration."

Lovers have a primary responsibility to each other, not to the standards of either the gay community or to society at large.

FINDING A PHYSICIAN

Gay men have special health problems that can be understood properly only by a doctor who has worked with and is sympathetic to gay patients. Many gay men insist on consulting with a gay physician because so many straight doctors are both ignorant of gay medicine and actively hostile to gay patients.

Some gay men have two doctors—one for their ordinary health problems and one for sexually transmitted diseases. This approach is irrational. Our bodies are not cordoned off into gay and straight zones. So-called gay health problems such as hepatitis, parasites, and venereal diseases may produce symptoms that will damage parts of your body not originally infected. It's best to have one doctor to keep track of all your health needs, and if you cannot come out to him or her and discuss your sex life and lifestyle, you need a different doctor.

How do you find a doctor sympathetic to the health needs of gay people? Gay service organizations and gay health clinics usually have a list of physicians. Some doctors even have health clinics with which they are associated. Friends will recommend doctors who have treated them competently. Gay health centers are listed in the *Gayellow Pages,* available in bookstores or by writing Renaissance House, Box 292, Village Station, New York, NY 10014.

You may, however, find yourself in a strange city (or country) and be unable to locate a gay physician. In that case you need to be able to tell a straight physician what you think may be wrong—especially if it's a sexual condition.

If a doctor you see refuses to treat you because you're gay, threaten to make a formal complaint against him or her with the local medical association. Of course you may not carry out the threat if you feel you must keep your own homosexuality a secret, but if you're already open about your homosexuality report him or her. A bit of gay militancy is in order when dealing with hostile straight doctors. For too long the health problems of gays have been neglected by irresponsible physicians.

Demanding your medical rights is extremely important if you or your lover is seropositive or symptomatic. There are still physicians and nurses who will treat you like a leper if you're ill. One hospitalized AIDS patient, for example, was visited by a house physician wearing work gloves and a paper bag over his head with eyehole slits. The doctor spoke to his patient from the threshold of the room. Needless to say, the patient recognized that he had a fool for a physician and immediately complained to the hospital administrator. Within an hour a new and competent physician was at his bedside. The moral? Don't take shit from a homophobe.

FIRST TIME

Throughout history men have fucked each other and relished the experience. They have persisted despite persecution by clergymen, judges, and doctors. This persistence in the face of such penalties as hanging, burning, castration, imprisonment, and commitment to mental hospitals indicates that fucking men and getting fucked is a great and enduring pleasure.

To get fucked and enjoy it, you may have to overcome some negative attitudes about your asshole (see *Anus*). The best preparation for getting fucked is to explore your anus and some of the sensations it can provide. Some men like to do the following exercises in a bathtub. The warm water helps you to relax, and the bathroom provides some privacy for young gay men who still live with their families.

Wash your anus, including just inside, with soap and water. Lubricate your finger with your preferred lubricant and insert it into your anus. As you feel increasingly relaxed, apply more lubricant and push deeper. You'll feel the sphincter muscles at this point; these need to relax for you to get fucked. Deliberately tighten them. You'll be surprised how strong they are. Relax them. Grip and relax these muscles several times.

Now move in deeper. You'll find the sphincter muscles are more extensive than you thought, and they open and relax of their own accord around your exploring finger. If they don't, don't try so hard.

Once your finger gets beyond the sphincter it enters the rectum, a wider space. You'll notice the change in texture. Move your finger in and out a couple of inches at a time. If you've been fearful about anal penetration until now, you'll be amazed how easy this is.

Remove your finger, breathe deeply, and relax. Tell yourself out loud that you're coming along beautifully. Complimenting yourself may seem absurdly narcissistic, but in fact it's a useful reinforcement, well known to behavioral psychologists. If after this break you insert your finger again, you'll notice how much more easily it goes in—but don't rush.

After several exploratory sessions, try two fingers. If you feel the sphincter muscles closing, return to the tightening and relaxing exercises. You may now use a dildo if the idea appeals to you. Make sure it's reasonably sized, and not one of those monsters that stunt artists absorb.

Two other exercises may be of value. First, if you have a fuck buddy or lover, ask him to explore your asshole with his fingers. Then put your fingers in his anus. The second exercise is that you jerk off with one hand while you insert one or two fingers of the other hand into your anus. As you masturbate, move your fingers rhythmically in and out. Again, you may want to invite your partner into the bathtub to perform these exercises with you. Given the close quarters, the session may end up both instructive and hilarious.

One note of caution. Fingers, dildos, and cocks can be pleasurable and are safe. *Never put anything else up your ass.* No glass bottles, sweet potatoes, or other exotic objects. They may elude your grasp, get lost in your intestines, and require major surgery (see *Sex Toys*).You should prepare in a number of ways for getting fucked the first time. Physically, all you need to do is to clean yourself out with an enema. You should also have condoms ready, and always insist your partner use them. We strongly advise you not to drink alcohol heavily or to use mind-altering drugs at this time. They may interfere with good judgment about safe sex (see *Booze and Highs*). Choose a lubricant that contains nonoxynol-9. Lubricate your asshole and the outside of your partner's condom liberally. You may also want to have your favorite jerk-off lubricant handy, to work on your own dick while getting fucked (see *Condoms; Lubricants; Safe Sex*).

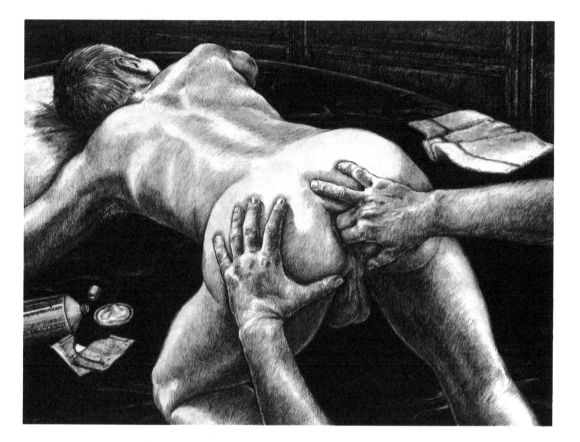

There are two good positions to start out with. The easier one involves both you and your partner lying on your sides, pitcher's front to catcher's back. Sometimes a novice will prefer to be on top so he can control the situation. In this position you face your partner, who is on his back, and you sit on his cock. Being on top will relieve what may be one of your main anxieties: that he will enter too quickly. If you are on top you can control the rate of penetration yourself, but remember that the average man can accommodate quite a large penis with no great difficulty. When his cock is about a third of the way in you may feel pain. Pull away gently and rest before trying again. The interval will give the sphincter time to open up.

On the second attempt, everything should go well. You should be able to accommodate the whole cock—in fact, you may be surprised how easily it goes in. If it doesn't, simply repeat the process, trying to relax.

The first few times you get fucked you may have the uncomfortable sensation that you are about to defecate. Only after several experiences will you learn to tell the two sensations apart.

Suppose you're finally at home with an attractive man you've been pursuing, and you're both undressed. Suddenly he announces that he's never been fucked before but wants to learn. Your reaction is crucial. Do you want to take on a novice? You may not be interested—or, on the other hand, you may be flattered. If you're not willing to take the time to do it right, skip it. Initiating a neophyte must be done patiently and carefully.

You must teach him to relax, guide him through clear, unambiguous instruction, reassure him that he's doing well, and never rush. Tense people are seldom aware that their bodies are rigid, their muscles contracted. Tell and point out to him where he's tense. Rub the spots, massage them a little. You don't have to be a professional to help him to feel good and relaxed (see *Massage*).

Enter him gently with one finger. After he's adjusted to one finger, enter with two—but not too quickly. Once you've got both fingers in his anus, masturbate him with your other hand. The familiar pleasure of masturbation, which he's known since puberty, is now linked with the new sensation of anal penetration. You could masturbate or suck him almost to the point of coming. Frustrate him a bit; make him wait for his climax.

You might want to have him do the same to you, and even reverse roles, taking turns jerking or sucking each other, until he's comfortable and hot.

Now you're ready to fuck him. Lets say he's on his back with his legs around your shoulders. While massaging his cock with your hand, explore his anus with the fingers of your other hand, then with the head of your cock. Asks how it feels. When he seems eager and fully relaxed, put the head of your cock in, but not entirely. Let him get used to the sensation before continuing.

The first entry should be slow and gentle. Partial entry is par for the course; don't try to force your way. If he tenses up, withdraw and use your fingers to massage his anus again. If he begins to panic, stop what you're doing. If you're partly or completely inside him, ask if he wants you to pull out. Say it in a calm way. Even begin to retract a little. *It's his body being invaded: Let him guide you.* Sometimes knowing that you can be trusted is enough to relax him.

Let him know what you're feeling—how exciting being inside him is, and how sexy and handsome he is. Continue to jerk him off, but not to the point of climax. Get him to vocalize what he's feeling: Vocalizing will help him feel pleasure (see *Dirty Talk; Noisemaking*).

Thrust slowly and gently. From time to time let him initiate the movement; vary his position until your penis massages his prostate—a sure site of pleasure. Finally, after you both come, kiss him, hold him, and tell him how good it felt to be inside him.

FISTING

Fisting is the insertion of the whole hand and wrist through the rectum and into the sigmoid colon. It is dangerous and can result in complications that lead to death. A sharp fingernail can leave a deep, painful cut in the rectum that could take weeks to heal. A fist ramming the sigmoid colon—the part of the intestine eight inches up from the anus—could be fatal.

The tissue lining the sigmoid colon has the consistency and delicacy of wet paper towels. In some cases it can expand to accommodate a closed fist, but internal bleeding can result, as can infection of the peritoneum (as well as the membrane lining the abdomen), and cause peritonitis. Since the bleeding is internal, it produces no visible blood. Some men have recognized the symptoms (stomach cramps, chills, and fevers) and rushed to a surgeon. A colostomy—rerouting of the intestine to a sac on the side of the body— saved their lives.

The harm done in fist-fucking comes about because there are no pain receptors in the intestines. The person being fisted can't tell what's going on inside him. Since a lot of fist-fucking occurs when people are high on drugs, physical sensitivity is reduced. Drugs may also interfere with good judgment (see *Booze and Highs; Drugs*).

Many gay men would consider this description unnecessarily alarmist and naive. Despite these obvious dangers, fisting was quite popular in the past, mostly among sadomasochists, and some of the best-selling porno films of the pre-AIDS era—*L.A. Tool & Die; Fists of Fury*—dealt with it in a most erotic manner.

The Fistfuckers of America, or FFA, assures us that there are numerous cases of men taking a fist with no apparent damage. Not all fisting depends upon pain and dominance. To take a whole hand requires such total relaxation that after getting fisted a man might feel great tranquillity.

Fisting often occurs as the culmination of a very intense session of sexual activity. Often the person getting fisted has already been fucked for a while by his partner's cock, and his rectal muscles are relaxed. The fister should coat his hand and forearm with a thick layer of lubricant (see *Lubricants*), and should apply more lubricant throughout the process. The fister ought to have previously removed rings and bracelets from his hand and trimmed his fingernails, sanding down rough edges. If the person about to be fisted notices that his partner's nails are long or sharp, he should insist they be trimmed there and then.

Fisting begins with the insertion of one or two fingers to loosen up the muscles; three or four fingers follow. The fister then pulls out his hand, folds his thumb against his palm, and wriggles his entire hand back in. The difficult part is getting the entire hand past the sphincter.

The man getting fucked will take whatever position facilitates entry. Some lie on their backs with their feet in the air; others crouch on all fours. Another position is to stand, then slowly sit on a vertical forearm.

A new problem has arisen with fisting: HIV Disease. Most researchers believe that HIV is easily transmitted through the blood-rich system of the anus, rectum, and colon. Any practice that causes trauma (damage) to any part of this area is therefore deemed an unsafe sexual practice. Some fisters try to minimize this danger by wearing a rubber glove during fisting, condoms when fucking, and by never ejaculating in the bottom's asshole. Still, fisting remains a questionable practice. And needless to say, you should not insert any dangerous object into your ass (see *Dangerous Sex*; *Sex Toys*).

FORESKIN

During the Roman Empire a foreskin was important cosmetically, to conform to ideals of beauty. Athletic games required competitors to have a foreskin that completely covered the glans penis (the head of the cock). But some athletes came from North Africa and the eastern Mediterranean, where circumcision was common. These athletes underwent an operation in which a new foreskin was surgically formed so that they could compete. With the fall of Rome, foreskin restoration stopped.

Circumcision originated among the ancient Hebrews as a way to mark their separateness from Gentiles. It is still practiced in the Jewish and Muslim religions, and throughout the United States by Gentiles. Sir Richard Burton, the English explorer, noted that some physicians believed circumcision discouraged masturbation, then called onanism. Circumcision became routine in the United States in the nineteenth century for the same reason. Today it serves no purpose (it certainly doesn't prevent masturbation), though it is frequently justified as a hygienic measure. A circumcised cock may be a bit easier to keep clean, but the uncircumcised need spend only a few seconds to be perfectly tidy.

Uncircumcised men occasionally claim that circumcision removes some sensitivity during sex, but one wonders how they know this. When erect, circumcised and uncircumcised cocks look and feel much the same.

Many gay men register strong preferences for "cut" or "uncut" meat; in fact, personal ads in gay publications often specify which is desired (see *Sex Ads*). For these men, the appearance of a partner's cock is probably an important factor in their fantasy life, though it limits the reservoir of potential partners. It's sad to think that men are rejected as sex partners or lovers because of a piece of skin.

We've met a few men who say that a foreskin is required for "docking": You place the head of your dick against the head of your partner's dick (face-to-face, so to speak). Then you pull his foreskin over both his dick head and yours—and you're docked. We have no idea what happens next. Perhaps a sci-fi scene? We should also note that some men like to place jewelry on their foreskins (see *Piercing*).

Sometimes medical circumcision is required on an adult man because the prepuce is too tight and prevents a full erection (this condition is called phimosis), or because of recurring infections. Circumcision among adults can be a serious and painful business and should not be undertaken for purely cosmetic reasons. Occasionally, men attempt to restore their own foreskins, or circumcise themselves without medical assistance. This can result in mutilation or serious infection.

FRIENDSHIP

Friendship means more to most gay men than it does to many straights, and gays learn how to value and cultivate it. Both straight and gay teenagers know the intimacy and ardor of friendship, but all too many straights "grow out of" those fierce involvements and pour all their emotional energies into their husbands or wives, and children.

Parents of gays often puzzle over how their children can endure the loneliness of single life. Since the parents are usually very rooted in their marriages and often receive little real sustenance from friends, they would naturally have difficulty understanding a life-style in which friendship is central. Typically, a gay man will have two or three close friends, male and female, with whom he shares his hopes and doubts about his job, his health, his emotional and spiritual growth, and his personal goals.

Exceptions abound, naturally; there are married straights who maintain intense, one-to-one friendships, and, conversely, gay couples who socialize only with other couples. Nevertheless, experience seems to suggest that gays, especially those without lovers or between affairs, enjoy friendships that are active, supportive, candid, and nurturing.

Friendship is not a substitute for love; it is its own province, one that some philosophers have considered a higher affection than love—higher because, at its best, friendship is free from the need to dominate, to possess, or to use. Because friendship *is* so crucial to the happiness of most gays, they should take pains to make it thrive. Nothing is more irritating (and self-defeating) than the gay man who drops his friends and goes into hibernation the moment he finds a new lover.

Compared to the glamour of a new passion, friendship may seem a mild pleasure, but it's a pleasure that endures and ripens. Friends should not be taken for granted. They should be selected with care, and their feelings regarded with sensitivity.

FROTTAGE

Rubbing against someone, while clothed or naked, to the point of climax is called frottage. Unpleasant, beady-eyed straight men—and not-bad-looking gay men, too—practice it standing up in crowded elevators, in rush-hour subways and buses, or waiting on line in front of theaters. Teenagers in the fifties and sixties did it to excess in the backseats of jalopies; it was called heavy petting by the media. It's also something two men can do together at home. Some even prefer it these days, because it's safe.

Sometimes it's called belly-fucking, or the Princeton rub. One lubricates one's partner's stomach, climbs on top and pumps away. If one's ass is out

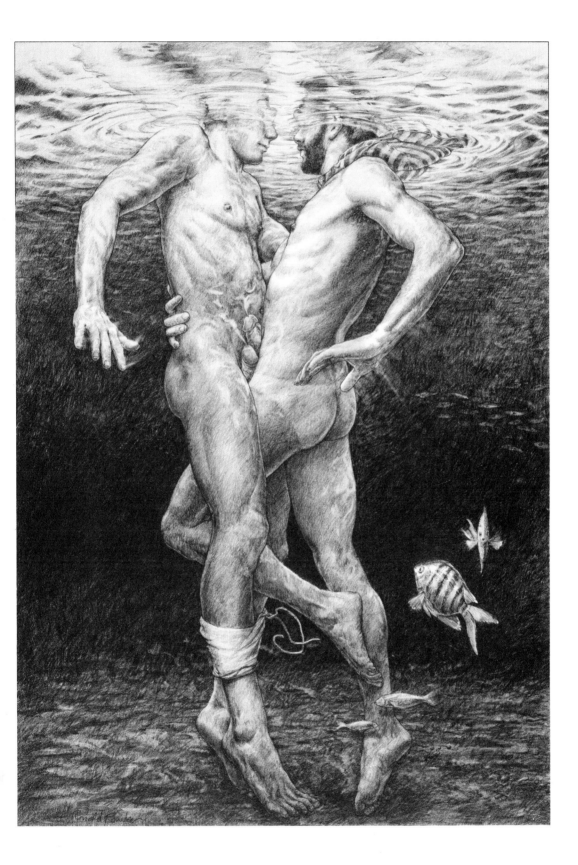

of commission for some reason, belly-fucking can be a good substitute, though it has appeals of its own and need not be considered a makeshift. Some men also like the feeling of rubbing their genitals against those of their partners until they come. If he's smooth-skinned between his legs, you can fuck the space between his thighs, just below his crotch (interfemoral fucking, as it's called). Armpits; the gully between the pecs; the crevice between the buns; the space between clavicle and chin when the head is tilted to one side are all similarly available. If you're wrestling, you can both rub against each other to the point of climax. You can even masturbate a cock with the soft soles of your feet.

FUCK BUDDIES

Let's say you meet someone new and the sex together is wonderful. The next time you meet in a club or bar, you go home again. After that, you bump into each other on the street, flirt, talk dirty, and end up having sex again. You exchange phone numbers and arrange for more sex. You're seeing each other regularly, having hot, satisfying sex, and you've come to look forward to these encounters. While the relationship is warm and affectionate, intuitively you both know you'll never become lovers. No problem; there's a perfectly good name for this common relationship in gay life—you're fuck buddies.

Having a fuck buddy means you can indulge your sexual fantasies without entangling alliances, and without the emotional turmoil of a romance. Of course, finding a compatible fuck buddy is as difficult as finding a lover. Looking for one doesn't work: It just happens. A good fuck buddy is perfect if you have no interest in having a more intimate relationship.

Use your fuck buddy to perfect your technical skills and to expand your repertoire. It's not unusual for someone to integrate new sexual skills discovered with a fuck buddy into his relationship with his lover. In this way, the relationship with the fuck buddy can help the relationship between two lovers.

Tops who want to be bottoms for a day, or vice versa; men who want to experiment with all the different kinds of fucking and sucking in this book; and guys who are interested in trying out kinkier stuff can do so freely as long as their fuck buddies agree (see *Sleazy Sex*).

The mutual pleasure of the fuck buddies is the quid pro quo of the relationship, with the implicit understanding that the relationship can be ended at any time with no hard feelings.

without much later effect, it was called the Society for Human Rights. Its goal was to educate the public about homosexuality and to repeal the sodomy laws. This organization was hounded by the police and the press, and soon driven out of existence. (Read *Gay American History* by Jonathan Ned Katy.)

The sexual climate in the United States was extremely difficult for homosexuals right up to and throughout the Second World War. They were subjected to arrest, entrapment, imprisonment, psychiatric and medical mistreatment, and legal castration.

The Second World War is considered by many sociologists and historians as the key event responsible for bringing out American lesbians and gay men. Huge numbers of young people were drafted or enlisted, taken off the farms and out of factories, thrown together in boot camps, on ships, in barracks, and allowed to socialize.

The publication of the Kinsey Report to a startled public in 1948 confirmed what many had already guessed: the widespread extent of male homosexuality in all levels of American society. Groups of gays began to meet, notably Harry Hays's pathbreaking (1950) Mattachine Society in Los Angeles, which published the first homosexual magazine, *ONE*. In 1955, the Daughters of Bilitis, a lesbian organization, was founded in San Francisco; its publication was *The Ladder*. When the U.S. Postal Service banned the distribution of an issue of *ONE* and pronounced any mention of homosexuality obscene, the ban was appealed. The Supreme Court decided in favor of the publication and against the post office—an important legal victory for gays. (Read *Making History: The Struggle for Gay and Lesbian Equal Rights, 1945–1990* by Eric Marcus.)

Even so, by 1969 there still were only about fifty gay organizations in the whole United States. Then a major, spontaneous upsurge of gay militancy occurred. On June 28, 1969, the New York City police raided and attempted to close a gay bar called the Stonewall Inn. For the first time (it had been raided often) the gay clientele—composed mainly of street hustlers and transvestites—actively resisted the police. Many of the cops were bludgeoned to the ground by the purses and high heels of the transvestites in the bar. The rebellion became so fierce that the police took sanctuary inside the bar, locking themselves in until reinforcements arrived.

It was an early summer night, a day after the funeral of the singer Judy Garland (a homosexual icon), and the nearby blocks were already filled with many gay residents who quickly joined in the mêlée, turning it into a major riot. The surrounding area in Greenwich Village was cordoned off and the riot squad brought in. By the next afternoon, a large picket line and protest rally had gathered at Sheridan Square. Overnight a new spirit was born, one patterned to some degree on the black civil-rights movement.

Two major organizations were founded out of the gay protest against police department policies; first the Gay Liberation Front and, after that failed, the more successful Gay Activists Alliance. The GAA, though committed to nonviolence, confronted discrimination at the risk of arrest. (Read *Under the Rainbow: Growing Up Gay* by Arnie Kantowitz.) They originated the "zap," a public demonstration using humor to highlight prejudice against gay people. In one zap they brought two wedding cakes to the New York City Marriage License Bureau, which had previously refused marriage licenses to two gay men and two gay women. On top of the cakes were the customary brides and grooms, except that there were two grooms on one cake and two brides on the other. While officials frantically phoned the police, gays from the GAA cut the cakes and handed slices to the office staff. There were no arrests, but lots of newspaper publicity—which, of course, was the goal of the zap. In another case, a member of the City Council was holding up passage of a gay-rights bill. Every Saturday night at three A.M. (after the GAA dance) about a thousand gay men marched to his apartment house and demonstrated in the streets, keeping him (and his neighbors) up for an hour or two. Thereafter, gay militancy became the order of the day, and activist groups were formed in almost all major American cities, each devoted to achieving civil rights for gay people.

Militant gay groups are still demonstrating against prejudice (see *Civil Rights*). This has become the primary goal of Queer Nation and of other groups, like the Gay and Lesbian Alliance Against Discrimination (GLAAD), which have targeted antigay attitudes and reportage in the media. ACT UP, another militant group, has devoted itself to only one agenda: fighting governmental inaction in AIDS research and treatment.

There are gay organizations all over the country—health services, self-help groups like the People with AIDS Coalition (PWAC), community centers, gay political clubs, legal services, and professional associations. Many are working to reverse discriminatory statutes, to educate the straight public about gay life, and to provide badly needed services for the gay community.

Unlike its predecessors, the American gay movement following the Stonewall riots became a "shot heard 'round the world," and responsible for the explosive growth of the gay-rights movement not only in the United States but internationally as well. Following the lead of American gays, Europeans, Asians, South Americans, and Africans have begun to come out.

GAY POLITICS AND POLITICIANS

Gay politics arose out of the Stonewall riots in Greenwich Village in, 1969. A number of gay-liberation organizations were formed soon after the riots. These included the Gay Liberation Front, the Gay Activists Alliance, and the National Gay Task Force. They had clearly defined goals. First, to secure freedom from harassment and arrest for gays who gathered in bars, restaurants, clubs, on the streets—in fact, anywhere. Second, to repeal any and all local, state, and federal legislation that criminalized homosexual acts between consenting adults. Third, to end the media's misrepresentation of all gays as effeminate, perverted, child-molesting, violent, and murderous.

To a greater extent than anyone thought possible at the time, these goals have been met—only partially, true, and only in selected cities and states, and always against a background of unceasing antigay prejudice and antigay activity by religious and political groups. Even so, given the short amount of time involved and the fact that other groups—women, African-Americans—have been fighting a century or longer for equality, gays have done well. The freedom of gays to associate is now a constitutional right, upheld even where prejudice is strongest. Half the states in the Union have repealed sodomy laws, and there is constant lobbying and legislative activity to repeal them throughout the nation. Virtually every large city in the country—except a few in the South—has done likewise. Today even counties and nonurban population centers are removing outdated, antigay laws on their books. And in southern California a few years ago, the community of West Hollywood broke away from the surrounding city of Los Angeles to become the first independent city in the United States with a majority of lesbian and gay residents, and a gay government.

Unfortunately, the one time a state sodomy law—that of Georgia—was brought to the Supreme Court, the judges upheld it even though Georgia's own attorney general has spoken out against it, refused to use it, and asked for its abolition. Also on the negative side, verbal "hate crimes" and physical violence against gays continue around the country—most disturbingly, on college campuses—and they seem difficult to stop legally.

While it has been an uphill battle and seems to be a never-ending one, the media have made great strides toward eliminating outright lies, slanders, insults, and the grossest misrepresentations of gays in their pages and on the airwaves. An entire new generation of media workers exists that—with one important exception—seems not only acclimated to this new order, but also sensitized to gay images and issues. The exception, of course, is the Hollywood film industry, which continues to ignore gay issues, or to present them only in the most bigoted, stereotypical terms.

Given all this, it's striking that so few national gay leaders have emerged. A few have come to prominence over the years, but as their organization or power base or the issue they were connected with either ended or was solved, they fell back into the ranks.

Strongly positive and useful as this political work has been in keeping the general gay and nongay population apprised of gay issues, much of the real work of gay politics is done not in the public's eye, but behind the scenes, in political party headquarters, in city hall corridors, in statehouse offices, in federal governmental department meetings and legislative committee rooms. It's there that laws are drafted, rules are changed, and important politicians are persuaded to make gay rights and gay issues part of their overall strategies. It's there that the grunt work is done to change antigay laws and to alter perceptions of gay life. But publicly, too, gay politicians are gaining ground, openly campaigning and winning seats on municipal councils, boards of supervisors, even boards of education; and also becoming state representatives and senators, even representatives to the U.S. Congress, which at the time of this writing has two openly gay members.

In the last few years, new issues have been added to the quiverful gay politicians already have to shoulder. Discrimination against gays in employment, housing, and medicine is one—and antidiscrimination laws are going on the books at city halls and even selected statehouses all over the nation. Equally important is the question of gays as parents, especially in custody cases and adoptions; it remains a crucial area for future legislation.

Above all, unfortunately, has been the overwhelming issue of AIDS, and how to legally secure and insure new life-extending drugs and procedures for the ill, as well as full medical and financial protection, social services, legal aid, hospitalization and hospice care, even the protection of last wills and testaments from antigay relatives (see *Insurance; Living Wills; Wills*). AIDS has proven to be a massive, all-fronts war, and gay politicians have been in the forefront, fighting for the rights of the sick. In the last few years, groups such as ACT UP and its offshoots have taken gay politics back to the activist days of the seventies, back into the streets, indeed into the very halls and apses of gay oppressors themselves in angry, often scandalous demonstrations that have galvanized the public's attention and as often polarized support and opposition.

One new and controversial subject in the gay community is "outing." The term means that a gay man (or lesbian) who has remained closeted— his gay identity unacknowledged even though it may be known to many people—is publicly called a homosexual in the gay press, and eventually the straight media. He can be in government, entertainment, or the arts, but the controversy over his sexual identity will always be on public record.

Those who out others do so because they believe the closeted individual has hurt the gay community through his or her hypocrisy and homophobia. By outing him they reveal this hypocrisy and self-hatred and reduce his ability to do further harm. Many who out public figures stop there, but some go further, outing people who may have never done any harm to gays. Usually, this kind of outing comes about during times of antigay sentiment or stress. The reason given to support this kind of outing is that every gay is needed to help the movement, or that every gay must stand up to show our strength and numbers.

Many gays oppose outing, calling it an invasion of privacy and a potential threat to a person's reputation and employment. This is true, although in the United States public figures have limited rights of privacy, and most public figures accept this as a by-product of fame.

Gay political leaders prefer that admired gay public figures come out so as to provide good role models to gay youth. (Recently a Marvel Comics hero, Northstar, "came out.") Despite this argument, and given our homophobic culture, outing is always a risky venture with unpredictable results.

In the years to come, that double-pronged effort—public, out in the streets, and private, behind closed doors in offices—will doubtless continue. It remains to be seen whether one or more gay politician in office, about to be elected or not yet on the horizon, will arise to become a national leader. If so, given the great range, variety, and especially the extremely critical bent of gays, he will have to be extraordinary—of impeccable politics and background, and with an already well-established stature—if he is to represent and lead (see *Civil Rights; Gay Liberation*).

GROWING OLDER

According to gay lore, "Nothing is sadder than an old queen." For young gay men who are thoroughly enjoying their sexual orientation, the prospect of growing old generates a great deal of anxiety: They nervously study the mirror for wrinkles and watch the approach of each birthday with dread.

The truth about aging is different. Studies have shown that older gay men are usually happier, more content, and better adjusted than younger gay men (which may be why some younger men prefer mature partners).

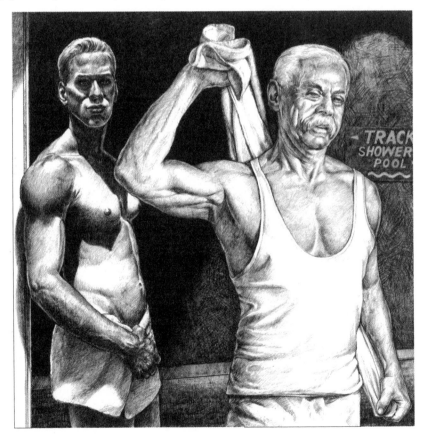

An older man has usually learned a lot about himself, has built a circle of friends, and has achieved a degree of success in his career; these can compensate for the physical changes brought about by age. (Read *Gay and Gray: The Older Homosexual Man*.)

Of course, there are men in their late fifties, sixties, and seventies who still incessantly cruise the streets or haunt the bars. They were probably always unhappy, even when they were twenty or thirty. Well-adjusted older gay men are simply not that visible in the "combat zone."

A successful older gay man recognizes that what he has to offer may not be immediately apparent. He may not look as dashing as he did when he was young, but with age he has become more secure, more honest, more interesting, and more interested. These qualities may not manifest themselves across a crowded room, but they show over the dinner table or in one-on-one encounters.

Quieter pleasures have superseded the more frenetic excitement of long nights at a club or the tortuous pursuit of a potential trick from bar to bar. The chase may still have its allure for an older man, but he generally knows how to conduct it with more patience, even more amusement, and if he is wise he stages it on his own turf.

Many mature gay men have been or are in long-lasting relationships. We've met couples celebrating their fiftieth anniversary. They live quiet, happy lives.

Straight or gay, older men almost always retain sexual desire and the ability to perform (if not with the same frequency). What's lost in firm muscle or dewy skin is replaced by much greater sexual technique, versatility, and sophistication. And if there is a diminution of sexual drive this may, paradoxically, lead to a greater sense of control. Young men are often so sexually driven they waste too much time trying to get laid, spending hours with people they may lust after but not like, whereas older men, having learned by experience, are better able to assess all the factors, control their desires, and select partners with more care. Senior Action in a Gay Environment (SAGE) is an organization for older gay men and women. Call its New York chapter (212) 741-2247 for information about a chapter near you.

GUILT

Guilt—in any number of forms—is a deep and persistent problem for homosexuals, and overcoming it is a long but fulfilling and liberating experience. Like the devil, as described by the Puritans, guilt insinuates itself into the most private corners of the heart and comes dressed in many clever disguises. Most of us feel that we are far too intelligent and sophisticated to be plagued by anything as old-fashioned and silly as guilt. But it's precisely the intelligent, sophisticated person who has the most difficulty in clearly labeling the guilt that haunts so much of his behavior.

Some gay men so disapprove of their own homosexuality that they hate themselves not just for what they *do* but for what they *are*. Often this sense of guilt is not experienced directly but masquerades as chronic depression. A person suffering from profound guilt believes he should be punished for . . . well, not for his wrong-doing but his wrong-*being*. Accordingly, he does nothing to stand up for his civil rights.

Most gay men, however, suffer from less severe forms of guilt. They feel guilty not for being, but for doing specifically "bad" things, which can range from cheating on a lover to experimenting with S/M and liking it. Or they may feel guilty about being gay—but only intermittently, when they read a condemnation of homosexuality in the press or when their parents look hurt and disappointed.

Guilt may be either conscious or unconscious, the latter being particularly hard to root out. It can manifest itself in excessive cleanliness, in excessive politeness, in a compulsion to work too hard. Unhappily, many gay men who suffer from internalized homophobia transfer their feelings of guilt to other gays and despise them as a substitute for hating themselves. Your guilty feelings may also be motivated by a desire to please your parents (see *Homophobia; Parents*).

In plumbing your guilt feelings, you may learn that lying just below your guilt about being gay is a more general guilt about sex of any sort. Some children are brought up in families where sex is bad, no matter what form it takes. The relationship between the parents is so poor that it leaves children with a sense of despair about all love relationships.

Guilt manifests itself in other aspects of gay life—compulsive cruising, inability to succeed in business, romantic fascination with straight men, an exclusive taste for quickie sex, or a penchant for "hopeless" love affairs with unobtainable partners. Guilt breeds a fear of intimacy and the self-contempt and longing for punishment that underlie so many of these behaviors. A more elusive expression of guilt is the desire to do endless favors for other people, to woo them in hundreds of little daily acts, to be a professional nice guy (see *Pleasure Trap*). This compulsion to please, usually linked to an inability to say no, often arises from a need to demonstrate that one is likable in spite of the terrible fact of one's being homosexual. Self-contempt endows the individual with an inexhaustible trust fund of guilt that can be drawn on by anyone and on any occasion.

The best way of overcoming guilt feelings about being gay is to participate with other gays in civil-rights organizations like ACT UP and Queer Nation. The object is to actively fight back against the institutions that made you feel guilty (see *Civil Rights; Depression; Gay Liberation*). The more conservative-minded person might work as a volunteer in an AIDS service organization. As long as a person is isolated from the gay community, he stands a much-reduced chance of dealing with his guilt feelings.

If participation in gay groups does not relieve feelings of guilt, then psychotherapy is recommended.

GYMS

Given the great emphasis Americans place on health and fitness, gyms have become increasingly popular. In fact, gyms have become to the nineties what bars and clubs were in previous decades: a basic, central location where gay men can meet and socialize. Though gyms aren't a sexual hangout, encounters do happen.

Before the 1970s, most gyms were straight-owned and straight-operated, functional spaces with wall-to-wall carpeting in shades of lime or mustard, with low ceilings and walls of mirrors. As a rule, they were located in urban downtowns or within ethnic middle-class enclaves and catered to off-duty policemen, firemen, the occasional boxer, and a few diehard bodybuilders. During that decade, especially following the success of the film *Pumping Iron,* bodybuilding became more respectable. The most famous straight gyms were the Mid-City, in Manhattan, and Gold's Gym, in Venice Beach ("Muscle Beach"), California. Gold's subsequently opened branches all over the country.

The earliest known gay gyms were small and attached to private homes or businesses in resorts such as the Fire Island Pines, Fort Lauderdale, and Laguna Beach. Spots such as Merrill's and the slightly more public Botel Gym at the Pines became crowded social gathering places on Saturday afternoons. Before every sizable party some men pumped up to maximum visual and tactile effect. Naturally, that was in the P.N.E., or Pre-Nautilus Era. Movable weights, not solid machines, formed the full selection of equipment, and it wasn't unusual to see someone step off the Sayville Ferry on a holiday weekend with luggage consisting entirely of a ton of dumbbells, barbells, weights and a paper bag containing a fresh T-shirt and a Speedo.

Nowadays, with a minimum of one gym per gay neighborhood, you can find guys working out to get or keep in shape, while they watch the latest video release or catch up on the latest gossip. On weekend afternoons the clientele can be as impolite as a rush-hour crowd on the Hollywood Freeway or the Lexington Avenue line as members angle in to get at those Nautilus machines, which promise perfect lats and deltoids to die for.

While most men rely only on physical exercise to increase their muscles, some also take steroids. The effect of these drugs, which are androgens (male hormones), is to increase the bulk of the body. In high doses, they cause high blood pressure and liver damage, including tumors of the liver. They also shrink the testicles. (This occurs because the testes don't need to produce androgens after they are artificially introduced into the body.) If you find yourself in bed with a man with big tits and small balls, you've taken home a steroid user. Tell him that the practice is medically unsound.

HAIR

Colette once said that long hair is a nuisance every moment of the day —except in the morning when making love. Then you can throw it forward, trail it across someone's skin, and (here one takes a step beyond Colette) look up through a dense curtain at your partner's eyes as you go down on his cock. But then, short hair has its charms as well—for though a buzz cut makes you look like a clipped cadet, to a lover it feels like a luxurious sable brush as you burrow your head in his armpit or crotch.

Almost every hairstyle has its erotic appeal, at least when viewed from a distance. Up close, however, hair brittle with gel or mousse can be unappetizing. If you've lost your hair, polish your dome and let it catch every light. Baldness is a forceful, masculine feature, especially to those who think that it results from an excess of male hormones. If you can't bear to be bald, then have those expensive and painful transplants, but don't wear a toupee or comb long strands across the barren desert—you'll be fooling no one.

Body hair also has its admirers. The Bear has lots of it (see *New Macho Images*). A sure sign of it is a tuft of hair showing at the collar or on the wrists.

Nothing is more versatile than hair. A full beard lends a saturnine (even satanic) look to the face, especially if the beard is precisely trimmed. Shaggier beards run the gamut from looking windswept and philosophical (old hermit in a mountain cave) to seeming robust and outdoorsy (lumberjack in town for a day to raise some hell). A droopy mustache can be poetic and deepen the eyes to spiritual pools; a neater, sharper mustache can turn you into an Edwardian roué. Some men insist upon a mustache on their partners; others recoil from facial hair as being unhygienic.

As you experiment you may find that with each change of hairstyle you attract a new class of admirers. Playing around with your facial hair is the main way you can modify the image you project. A pretty boy bored with a world of doting daddies who consider him cute can transform himself into a tough punk by growing his beard for three days, cutting his long locks, or shaving his head almost to the skin. A middle-aged hunk with a beard, a bald head, and a leather jacket, weary of having tricks ask him to piss on them or burn their chest, can attract respectable types by shaving and dressing in a jacket and tie (see *Shaving; Types*).

Naturally hairstyle fashions change every decade: The bearded or at least mustached ''clone'' of the seventies vanished by the mid-eighties and was replaced by a more classic, fifties look, with no hair on the face. Who knows? That look may be gone in a few years, too.

HANDS

Since the hands are our most sensitive nongenital equipment, precisely coordinated and packed with nerve endings, they can be used to perform the most delicate work. They can make feathery, just noticeable contact with the down on another man's body—especially the tiny hair above the tailbone, along the nape, around the nipples, on the insides of his thighs, and on his balls.

To appreciate the pleasure hands can give: Lie beside your partner and kiss him, but don't let any other parts of your bodies come into contact; as he becomes more excited, trail your fingertips over the sensitive flesh of his stomach. Pull back from the kiss and lightly trace the outlines of his mouth with your finger. Explore the inside of his mouth with your fingers, especially the front of the gums and the roof. Reach down and slowly trigger the hair on his balls. Wet your hands with your saliva and draw two lines on his stomach beside his penis (without touching it). Then graze his penis with your hand.

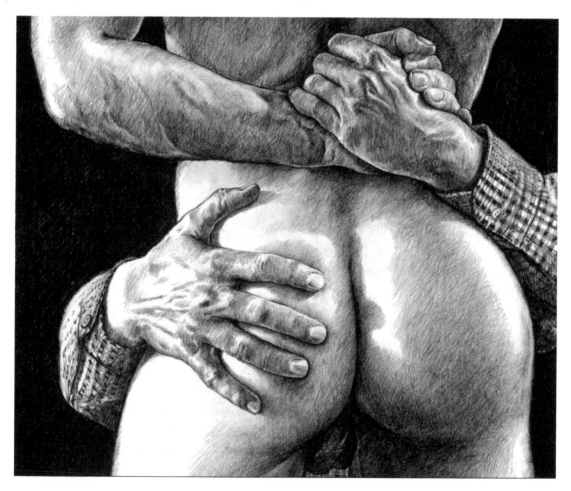

Hands can also stimulate other parts of his body, playing with his asshole, stroking his thighs and the backs of his legs, rubbing the bottoms of his feet, or pinching his nipples.

Remember, as your partner becomes more excited he can tolerate and will enjoy slightly rougher touching. When he gets sweaty and comes close to a climax, stop for a breather. As he calms down, blow a cooling stream of air over his sweaty body and follow this jet trail with light motions of your fingertips. While you're sucking him or he's fucking you, you can stick a finger up his ass to give him an extra sensation he will find exquisite. (He'll have a stronger climax, too.) Or you can reach under and grab his balls while he's fucking you; some guys like their balls to be pulled hard.

In rough sex, hands can make a vital contribution. You can pin your partner's wrists to the mattress as you fuck his face. You can squeeze his tits hard or slap his ass. And when all is done, you two can just lie there, exhausted, bodies too sore or overstimulated to touch, with hands entwined.

From the moment you first connect and your hands meet and begin to know each other at a bar, on a beach, or across a candlelit table, to the end of lovemaking, hands communicate and elaborate the language of love (see *Touching and Holding*).

HIV DISEASE

I n the early 1980s it was called GRID, for Gay-Related Immunodeficiency. Then the name was changed to AIDS, for acquired immunodeficiency syndrome. The federal Centers for Disease Control (CDC) is now considering a name change to HIV Disease.

"HIV" stands for "human immunodeficiency virus," the virus believed to cause the disease—a virus responsible for the death of many thousands of gay men, and killing many thousands of other people as well. The name changes do not suggest confusion on the part of the CDC, a governmental organization charged with charting the progress (epidemiology) of all diseases. Rather they represent advances in understanding the nature of this epidemic and the means to challenge it. The terms "AIDS" and "HIV Disease" are used interchangeably throughout this book.

The following is the minimum you should know about HIV Disease. There are books written to assist your understanding of the disease and your part in either containing or spreading it. Some of these emphasize traditional medical treatments, while others recommend alternative or holistic treatments. (Read *The Caregivers' Journey: When You Love Someone with AIDS* by Mel Pohl and Deniston Kay.) And since information and treatment are progressing rapidly, some information contained here may rapidly become out-of-date. It is your responsibility to keep abreast of the latest research and treatment by reading the best gay periodicals available and by getting on the mailing list of gay and AIDS service organizations.

What Causes HIV Disease?

Medical authorities believe that a specific virus or group of closely related viruses causes the disease, and that this virus is transmitted mainly by blood and semen. Some (but not all) medical researchers also suggest that there are contributory causes of the disease. By this they mean that the infecting virus cannot harm you significantly unless some other specific germ or medical condition is also present. They think this because some men who are HIV positive come down with serious illnesses very quickly, while others remain asymptomatic (free of symptoms) for a decade or longer. They think the first group of men had the germ (or contributory cause) that activated the virus in their bodies, but the second group did not. We do not conclusively know if HIV works alone or in the presence of another germ. What we do know is that people in good health remain so for a longer period of time than those who abuse their bodies with drugs, alcohol, and untreated medical conditions. For instance, some gay men whose blood was frozen when they participated in a hepatitis study in the mid-1970s have learned (seventeen years later) that they were seropositive when the blood was taken, yet many still haven't developed symptoms.

No one knows how HIV originated, or where. Some believe it is a new disease in the world and others that it remained confined to one geographically inaccessible area until modern transportation gave it the opportunity to spread.

Should I Be Tested?

There is no reliable blood test to demonstrate the presence of the virus in the body: What we have is a test that shows the presence of *antibodies* against the virus in your blood. Those who have the antibodies are said to be *HIV-positive* or *seropositive*.

During the early days of the epidemic very few gay men were tested because the tests weren't very accurate, and because there were few treatments available, and even those were ineffective. Gay-liberation organizations maintained that early diagnosis was useless in the face of ineffective treatment. There was also a justified fear that homophobic municipalities and states would collect lists of HIV-positive people and use them to discriminate against gay people (see *Civil Rights; Gay Liberation; Insurance*). It is in the nature of homophobes to blame gay men for the disease instead of recognizing that we are its victims. Homophobic politicians once proposed that HIV-positive men and AIDS patients be involuntarily placed in special camps, called isolation camps by homophobes, and concentration camps by gays.

Times have changed. There have been medical advances in the treatment of the various diseases caused by HIV, and virtually all gay organizations now recommend that sexually active gay men be tested for the presence of HIV *antibodies*. However, they suggest that counseling be included in the testing process so you can be aided both medically and emotionally if the test is positive. Also, the very act of testing can be upsetting to some people. Many municipalities now provide anonymous testing either through your own physician or through local clinics. You should consult with local gay organizations to determine the best way to be tested in your area, even if you should be tested, so that the information will not be transmitted to insurance companies, governmental agencies, or employers.

Despite these recommendations, the question of whether or not to be tested remains one only you can answer. You should be prepared for a major alteration and change of focus in your life—from whatever it has been, to an emphasis upon your health. Naturally, if you believe that you have symptoms of the disease, or if any of your sex partners have developed the illness, you should be tested.

If you test HIV-positive, your physician will want to do another test to check your *T-cells*. The T-cells are also called T-4 or CD4 helper cells. They are an important ingredient in the immune system, which protects the body from disease. A normal T-cell count runs anywhere from 600 to over 1,000. However, the count can temporarily go down whenever you are ill or fighting off a bug of some kind, and it may also vary widely during the day. It's therefore best to get T-cell testing when you're neither acutely ill nor sick with an infection.

Testing positive is not the same thing as having HIV Disease. It only means that you have been exposed to the virus and that antibodies have formed in reaction to its presence. The *diagnosis* of AIDS means that a person has come down with specific illnesses.

How Is Someone Diagnosed?

HIV Disease is diagnosed in one of two ways. The oldest way is the presence of HIV-related illnesses, usually called *opportunistic infections,* because they have taken the opportunity of immunosuppression to attack the body. (A list of such infections follows.) Modern medicine, however, has been somewhat successful in preventing and controlling many HIV-related illnesses. Therefore, the Centers for Disease Control is proposing to diagnose HIV Disease in any person with fewer than 200 T-cells, even in the absence of HIV-related symptoms. This means that many gay men who are technically asymptomatic will be diagnosed with HIV Disease, making them eligible for certain kinds of disability insurance and other medical and/or financial help. Everyone diagnosed should seek advice about eligibility from an AIDS service organization.

What Are the Symptoms?

There are a variety of early symptoms of HIV Disease, but none are unique to AIDS: All can also exist in the absence of the virus. Therefore, don't diagnose yourself if you happen to have one or more of these symptoms: It may be caused by a completely different and less dangerous virus or bacterium. Here's a short list of the most common minor symptoms.

1. *Swollen lymph nodes* most often occur first under the jaw. There is no pain, and no treatment is necessary or available.

2. *Night sweats* during sleep. Night sweats are not just perspiration from being overblanketed; your pajamas and sheets will be soaking wet. There is no pain, and no treatment.

3. *Thrush* is a yeast infection. White patches appear in the mouth and on the tongue. The mouth feels sore as thrush spreads, and in an advanced stage the infection can move down the throat and into the esophagus and upper lungs, causing considerable discomfort. Severe cases make swallowing painful and difficult, and thus make food unappetizing and difficult to get down. Treatments are available that make thrush mostly an irritation rather than a danger; it's controllable in most cases.

4. *Hairy leukoplakia* are raised white discolorations under the tongue. They are not painful, but can disturb eating, at a time when gaining weight may be crucial. Treatment is satisfactory.

5. *Shingles* is a painful, blistering rash, generally on the legs or lower back, or around the hips. Since it is caused by a herpes-type virus—the same thought to be present in chicken pox—the rash follows a nerve in a bandlike formation. Treatment is available, both for the pain and for the rash itself, though it will still take two or three weeks for the rash to disappear, and there may be scarring.

6. *Seborrheic dermatitis* is a dry, scaly rash on the eyebrows, scalp, and sides of the nose. It is not painful, and treatment is excellent.

7. *Unexplained weight loss and fevers*. This is a catch-all category, and is the reason why HIV is known as Slim Disease in Africa. There are no specific treatments for these symptoms, unless lab tests show they are related to a specific disease. They are generally thought to be the direct result of the virus, rather than of an opportunistic infection.

The most important major illnesses include:

1. *Pneumocystis carinii pneumonia (PCP)*. This used to be the major cause of death in AIDS patients. In the absence of HIV testing, it was often the first indication of illness in the infected person. It is now somewhat more preventable, and is treatable when it occurs. Whereas formerly PCP meant long hospitalization, now it is commonly treated by a variety of potent new drugs. Prevention of PCP is now a regular part of HIV Disease treatment. Many receive biweekly or monthly prophylactic inhalants on an outpatient

basis. Symptoms of PCP include high fever; a dry, nonproductive (no phlegm) cough; a progressive shortness of breath, particularly when exerting oneself; and searing knifelike pains in the back and joints.

2. *Kaposi's sarcoma (KS)* ordinarily manifests itself as dark, cancerous spots that can appear anywhere on the body. At first they are bright purple; then they turn deep brown or almost black. KS is not considered life-threatening unless it invades organs inside the body. In fact, for unknown reasons, when KS occurs in the absence of any other opportunistic infection, it is often associated with greater longevity for the AIDS patient. KS lesions can be very unsightly when they spread over the skin, and while not painful at first, they can be very sensitive to touch and pressure later in the disease process. There are local treatments for more extensive KS. New treatments are in the testing stage. However, no therapies are curative.

3. *Toxoplasmosis* is a protozoan infection of the brain. Symptoms include very high fever, severe headache, trouble with one's speech, and asymmetric (on one side of the body only) muscle weakness and sometimes convulsions. Toxoplasmosis progresses quickly (even hour by hour), so speedy diagnosis and treatment are crucial. One can be easily tested for the risk of acquiring the disease. Treatment is very good. The protozoan responsible is found in undercooked meats and used cat-litter-box filler.

4. *Cryptococcal meningitis* is an infection of the membranes that cover the spinal cord. As with toxoplasmosis, one can have fevers and headaches, but the patient may also experience neck stiffness, which is not a symptom of toxoplasmosis. Treatment is good if the infection is caught early.

5. *Dementia,* when it occurs, is one of the late signs of the disease. There are a number of symptoms, including shortness of memory (particularly recent memory), psychomotor troubles, difficulty with walking, loss of spontaneity and outside interests, a generally depressed mood (dementia is sometimes misdiagnosed as depression), and sudden extreme shifts in mood from extreme cheer, even exaltation, to the deepest despair. There are no treatments to reverse the damage to the brain.

Herpesviruses and HIV Disease

Herpes is a family of viruses that cause a number of illnesses from cold sores to shingles. The herpesvirus group also includes cytomegalovirus (CMV) and Epstein-Barr virus (EBV). None of them cause HIV Disease. On the other hand, HIV may *activate* dormant herpesviruses in those men who are infected with them, and the sleeping dogs of CMV and EBV may awake to bring considerable harm to the body, further weakening an already compromised immune system. The symptoms are subtle; there may be none, or the infected person may suffer flulike illnesses. Of course, not everyone has been exposed to herpes, and therefore not everyone with HIV Disease will have complications due to herpes. There are easy tests to diagnose herpes, and a variety of treatment is available.

It might also be added that a number of common illnesses become harder to treat in the presence of HIV Disease. The most important of those is syphilis, another reason to practice safe sex.

HIV Disease itself cannot be cured at this time. There are antiviral treatments available—the most common are AZT, DDI, and DDC—but they are all palliatives, meant to keep the virus at bay for a period of time. There is even a school of thought that suggests using them alternately, or one after another.

For more specific information, write to GMHC, (Gay Men's Health Crisis), 129 West 20th Street, New York, NY 10011. Ask for a copy of "Medical Answers about Aids."

(See *Body Positive; Mixed-HIV Couples; Sexually Transmitted Diseases.*)

There are four excellent newsletters available about AIDS treatment. They will reduce their subscription rates for people with low incomes. Sample copies are usually available at your request.

PWAC Newsline, published monthly by People With AIDS Coalition, free to PWAs, otherwise $30 a year, 31 West 26th Street, New York, NY 10010, 212-532-0290, Hot line 800-828-3280. This newsletter is written by and for PWAs.

Treatment Issues, published monthly by GMHC (address above), $30 a year, 212-337-1950.

AIDS Treatment News, published twice monthly by John S. James, $100 a year, PO Box 411256, San Francisco, CA 94141, 800-TREAT 1-2.

Project Inform, published monthly by Project Inform, donation of at least $25, 1965 Market Street, Suite 200, San Francisco, CA 94103, 800-822-7422.

HOMOPHOBIA

Why have homosexuals been persecuted and despised for centuries? What is the basis of homophobia (the fear of homosexuality)? There are three major theories. One holds that our society is sexually repressed and that homophobia is only one aspect of a more general condemnation of sexuality. While most people would agree that Western society is repressive, the theory does not explain why gays have been singled out with such particular animosity.

A second theory, derived from Freud, holds that we are all born bisexual, with the capacity to respond erotically to members of either sex. The homophobe, according to this theory, is the person who has not come to grips with his own latent homosexuality, who has neither adequately repressed nor accepted it. Instead of hating himself, the homophobe turns his anger against other homosexuals—a classic case of "projection."

The third theory is more recent. Research by social psychologists suggests that homophobia crops up in a society that maintains a strict distinction between male and female roles, especially one that assigns power and high status to men and dependence and low status to women. Gay people are feared and hated because they are perceived as challenging this distinction, muddying the otherwise pure, clear waters of gender-linked behavior. A gay man who could enjoy all the privileges of masculinity (respect, a good job, legal and economic superiority) is seen as willfully and perversely throwing away these advantages and embracing the lower status of a woman. Conversely, lesbians are seen as wanting to usurp male privileges. All the stereotypes invented by the straight world to punish gay people (the sissy faggot, the mannish lesbian) are designed to protect a breakdown of gender distinctions and of the unequal and unfair world of power, status, and wealth they represent. We can call this the *Gender Theory of Homophobia,* as it says that homosexuality as a social role rather than as a sexual practice is what upsets some straights.

It's ironic that society should define homosexuality as deficient masculinity. History is replete with examples of gay (or bisexual) military leaders who were every bit as capable as straight generals in the supposedly masculine arena of brutality and conquest. Julius Caesar, Alexander the Great, General Gordon of Khartoum, and Lord Kitchener all had male lovers.

There was a time when gay liberationists were sensitive to questions about the masculinity of gay men. We used to say that gender identity (our feeling of maleness or femaleness) was independent of our sexual identity (gay or straight). Like the society around us, we didn't want to be identified as deficient men—or, to put it another way, perceived as being like women. Although we didn't know it then, we were still identifying with society's concept of masculinity, and we chastised effeminate gay men for not being masculine enough.

There are many gay men who feel comfortable that their personalities contain both masculine and feminine components. There are gay men who feel the feminine side is the stronger and who go out of their way to nurture it. One also finds androgynous gay men expressing maleness or femaleness according to the occasion. Deprecating any of them is homophobic, whether the put-down comes from another gay man or from someone straight (see *Effeminacy*).

We believe that the *Gender Theory of Homophobia* outlined above best explains the hatred much of straight society has toward gay men and women. In fact, we believe it also explains *internalized homophobia*. The self-hating homosexual hates himself because he feels deficient as a man, and his self-hate is projected upon all other gay men. He can have sex in the dark or admire the masculinity of straight men, but he will be incapable of establishing an intimate relationship, because it will mirror his hatred for himself (see *Guilt; Pleasure Trap; Straight Men*).

Self-hating homosexuals are in a state of emotional conflict. Guilt plunges them into an "approach-avoidance" pattern, as psychologists call it. As they approach a lover, get to know him, they are happy and hopeful. But once the affair looks as though it might work, they back away and avoid the beloved, because the intimacy upsets them. As they withdraw, they breathe a sigh of relief, glad to be rid of this latest entanglement . . . but then they are once again alone and miserable. Loneliness drives them to attempt a new affair, with the same disastrous results. These dynamics are seldom expressed at the conscious level of a person's life. There's always something wrong with the new lover: He's lousy in bed; he's too young, too old, too extroverted or introverted. But the real reason such a man rejects his lover is self-hate for not being the man his parents (and society) demanded that he be.

HUSTLERS

There are all sorts of male prostitutes, commonly known as hustlers. Some make hustling a full-time profession, while others do it part-time, on nights and weekends, to supplement their income. Some work the streets and hustler bars; others meet clients through escort services, or advertise in gay publications. Hustlers hired off the street are potentially the most dangerous, whereas those hired through a service are generally the most reliable (also often the most attractive and expensive). All male prostitution is, of course, illegal in the United States.

Why do people hire hustlers? Sometimes they're in search of a kinky and hard-to-arrange scene (rubber, or the enactment of a highly detailed fantasy). If the scene is particularly elaborate or off-the-wall, hustlers will charge more. Others hire hustlers because they want a specific type (a small blond with a small cock, say, or a hairy man with a big cock) or they want to perform specific sexual acts (the small-cocked blond must fuck them, say). The point of hustlers is that one can fulfill a fantasy. A tall, masculine-appearing man may have a secret yearning to be thoroughly dominated, but in bars he is typecast as a "stud." By hiring a hustler, he escapes others' projections and satisfies his desires.

Hustlers are also employed by people too busy or too famous to cruise, as well as by tourists, businessmen at meetings and conventions, and married or bisexual men looking for some excitement. And then there are those johns (as men who hire hustlers are called) who are more turned on by paying for sex than by getting it free.

Many johns strike defensive postures (usually after sex). A john might insult the hustler overtly or covertly; tell him he never hired a "whore" before; attempt to impress with his superior wealth, intelligence, and connections. Hustlers are familiar with these strategems.

An encounter with a hustler can be pleasurable and civilized if each partner recognizes what can be gained from the experience—and what cannot: The john can forget love and companionship, and the hustler shouldn't expect a lifelong patron or an all-understanding father.

Hustling isn't easy. It takes mental and physical stamina to be able to deliver the sexual goods night after night. Many hustlers are permanently stoned on alcohol, grass, or downers. Others, especially those who begin hustling as young teens, can be left with deep psychological scars: alienation from their own bodies and distrust of affection. The work can also be physically dangerous.

Gay liberation changed the sales pitch of hustlers. Instead of presenting themselves as straight, today most hustlers admit they're gay and do anything the client likes.

Think twice before hiring a hustler. A few are angry, desperate, even psychotic; every year gays are killed by hustlers, though the numbers are probably no greater than murders occurring as a result of having sex with strangers. As you might expect, some hustlers are HIV positive or suffering from AIDS yet won't divulge the information because they need the money. If you must use a hustler, find someone reputable: Hire him through people you know or, better yet, call an escort service. Their business depends upon your safety—and pleasure.

Some men are aroused by the fantasy of being a hustler and play it out with sex partners. This seems like harmless fun to us.

IMPOTENCE

Every man has a problem with impotence from time to time. Perhaps the worst part of the problem is our embarrassment discussing it. We hide it the best we can.

Of course, impotence can't be hidden in the bedroom. When the clothes come off, the failure to raise and maintain a hard-on becomes painfully obvious. That's when men start looking for reasons. They blame alcohol, drugs, something they ate, fatigue, even the partner. Although there may be truth to some of these explanations, by and large they are excuses employed to alleviate feelings of humiliation. These are examples of situational, not chronic, impotence.

Before you decide you have a problem with impotence, ask yourself a few questions. Is the impotence intermittent or occasional? If so, don't worry. Everyone experiences variations in sexual performance, and an isolated or sporadic bout with an uncooperative dick may mean nothing more than that you weren't really turned on to your partner, that you had too many other things on your mind that night, or that you are coming down with an illness. An excess of alcohol and drug use almost always affects

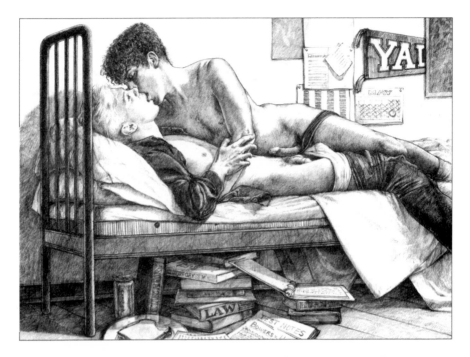

sexual functioning, and may cause temporary impotence as well (see *Booze and Highs; Drugs*).

However, repeated episodes of erectile failure increase the tension surrounding sexual activities. "Am I going to get it up?" becomes so anxiety-producing a fear that avoiding sexual contact is preferred to failure. Humiliation turns to hopelessness.

Psychoanalysis used to be the treatment of choice for impotence, for analysts believed that impotence was a psychological problem stemming from unresolved conflicts about one's parents or family. It was most often an ineffective course of action.

With the rise of sex therapy in the 1970s, treatment moved from deep analysis to direct behavioral intervention. Sex therapists believed that erectile dysfunctions developed because of inappropriate habits or attitudes about sex. They claimed that 80 percent of impotence was caused by psychological factors, and only 20 percent was due to physical causes. But the sex therapists were no more successful than the psychoanalysts.

In the last few years there's been a revolution in the treatment of impotence. Today, our best guess is that 80 percent of impotence has a physical origin, and only 20 percent is psychological. The newest theory suggests that impotence may be caused by a chemical imbalance of nitric oxide in the body, but the study that suggested this hasn't yet been replicated in other laboratories. Diagnostic procedures must be used to distinguish between physical and psychological erectile problems.

A few hospitals have erectile-dysfunction clinics, usually as a unit of the urology department. The clinic staff will take your sex history, give you a physical examination, and check your hormone levels. After that, a set of special tests is administered, using highly sophisticated equipment. First, you are given a computerized gadget to take home and put around your cock when you go to sleep. It's like a cock ring, and it measures the number of hard-ons you have while you sleep and how rigid your cock gets with each one. This is the single best test available to distinguish between physical and psychological impotence. If it's a physical problem, you will have fewer, less rigid erections during the night. If this is the case, and the origin of the impotence is physiological, a second test is performed.

The second test is a pharmacological screening. A drug injected into the cock produces a roaring hard-on. How long it takes to get hard, how hard it gets, and how long it stays hard give the doctor a good idea of whether the problem is arterial or venal in character.

Let us explain how a cock gets hard. When the brain sends a signal, blood rushes into the penis. It arrives by means of the arteries, and remains in your cock because the veins leading out are shut tight. The fluid pressure thus created makes your dick hard.

Three problems can occur in this process. First is the problem of nerve conduction, and here diabetes is the most frequent cause. Unfortunately, most physicians don't discuss impotence when diagnosing diabetes because they're uncomfortable talking about sex. The second problem involves arterial deficiencies. Special tests—invasive procedures, requiring injections —were developed to measure these, though they are now being diagnosed through the use of ultrasound. First, the doctor measures the arteries in your cock with an ultrasound machine. Then the roaring hard-on medication is injected into your cock and a second ultrasound picture is taken, measuring the ability of the arteries to expand and deliver blood.

Leaky veins in the cock lead to the third type of problem. In order to identify leakage, doctors inject a dye into an artery in your dick, and use X rays to track the progress of the dye through the veins.

A number of treatments are currently available, and some require surgery. The only noninvasive treatment, a vacuum restricting device, is actually a scientifically designed cock ring; it can help some patients. Of the invasive treatments, the mildest is self-administered. Just before sex, you inject a drug that produces a hard-on (an ultrafine needle is used). The more drug you inject, the longer the hard-on lasts, up to ninety minutes. The sexual sensations with the drug are just like normal. Some men get a bit upset with the idea of the injections, but the technique works. Use a bit of imagination. Perhaps you and your lover can play doctor!

The other physical treatments available today are far more invasive. Many urologists have joined the prosthesis bandwagon. A prosthesis is a surgical implant inserted into the cock. Implants have been used for a decade with mixed results. The newest design consists of a self-contained pump and reservoir. The pump is in the head of the cock; when you squeeze it, fluid is forced into the shaft and produces an erection. The release valve is also in the head of the cock. In another design, the "fully inflatable," the pump is placed in your balls and the reservoir of fluid in the abdomen. You get a hard-on when you squeeze your balls.

Other operations are being perfected by urologists. By means of micro-surgery, leaky veins can be tied off, and blocked arteries opened up. But the truth is that all of these procedures are still in an early stage of development. So the question is, Do they work? These treatments are so new that there aren't yet reliable statistics on their success rate. It can be a dreadful experience to complete testing and surgery, only to find one's dick as limp as before. Obviously, the least physically invasive procedures are the most reversible. If an implant doesn't work, you cannot reverse the damage done to your cock by the surgery.

We recommend that you have an evaluation and take the "cock ring" test that measures hard-ons during sleep. That will give you a good idea of how much of your problem is physical and how much psychological. If the test shows that your problem is psychological, get into therapy with a professional who respects your gay sexual life.

If the problem turns out to be physical, don't jump into surgery, no matter what any surgeon says. You'll need a lot of discussion with other professionals before you begin such invasive procedures. First, consult with your personal physician. If you can't talk to him or her about your sexual problems, get another doctor. Second, find a competent psychotherapist with whom you can discuss your feelings about sexuality. It's important that your therapist maintain a good working relationship with both your personal physician and the sex clinic. The therapist should be someone who will stand by you after surgery and guide your progress.

Counseling, before and after surgery, serves an important function. Some men blame all their social and romantic problems on not being able to get a hard-on. They sometimes fantasize that when they're restored to full sexual functioning, their lives will be magically transformed. They conjure up idyllic love relationships and marital bliss. But there's no magic in treating sexual dysfunctions. Even when surgery is successful, the hard work of establishing and maintaining a love relationship remains, with all the joys and pains that accompany the search for intimacy. The counseling procedure is crucial in helping a patient separate his physical problems from his search for love.

Of course all men want to perform well in bed. It's every bit as valid to want to overcome one's impotence so as to have a good fuck as it is to want a long-lasting love relationship. Sometimes sex is about passion. At other times it's lust and excitement we crave. We should function well in either situation.

INSURANCE

Learning about insurance may seem such a bore. This is especially true for those gay men fortunate enough to be automatically insured by their employers. But some of us are required to buy our own insurance because our employer doesn't provide it, or we're self-employed, or we've been laid off from a job. Gay men who are HIV-positive obviously have special needs and interests in the matter.

There are three kinds of insurance we need to discuss. The first is medical and dental insurance, which pays doctor and hospital bills; it may also cover office visits, home visits, or surgery. The second type is disability insurance, which pays a monthly stipend if you are temporarily or permanently unable to work. Finally, there is life insurance, which upon your death pays a specified sum of money to your beneficiary.

When you are first applying for a policy, most insurance companies ask questions about your past and current health, and seek permission to obtain further information from your physician. You may also be required to undergo a medical examination conducted by one of the insurance company's physicians, or to consent to take a blood test, which may include a test for HIV.

Insurance companies don't like to insure what they call preexisting conditions. That means any illness or medical condition you suffered from before your application or are still suffering from. Sometimes they will refuse to cover a particular illness altogether. For instance, virtually all insurance companies refuse to insure anyone who tests HIV-positive, while some others will not insure people with cancer or heart disease. Other companies may require a "waiting period," during which you cannot have coverage for a preexisting illness, but after which you'll be covered. Furthermore, some insurers won't pay for medicines and treatments that are "experimental"—even if the treatment is the only one that may save your life. If you work for a very large employer, the group policy may stipulate that all preexisting conditions will be covered immediately. You have to read the insurance booklet provided by your employer.

People always wonder whether they should lie about their medical history. "What's it their business?" some gay men ask. This is a complicated question for a number of reasons. Obviously, we can't recommend that you lie on insurance forms, since it's against the law. If you lie about your medical condition on the insurance application, then make a claim for doctor or hospital payments—and the insurer finds out you lied to them—it can claim fraud, and refuse to pay. The company may even cancel your insurance.

The problem of coverage for preexisting conditions is delicate. You need to have a good relationship with your personal physician and take an active part in your treatment by discussing the medical diagnoses he writes on insurance forms. It's also advisable to seek the counsel of a sympathetic insurance agent who can advise you.

One factor that makes discussing insurance so complicated is the variation of state laws governing such policies. Some insurance is governed by federal statutes, as well. It's important to search out a local gay or AIDS service organization so as to inquire about the laws in your state. They can probably recommend insurance agents and/or attorneys who specialize in getting insurance for gay people. Listen to what they have to tell you, because the laws controlling insurance change frequently.

A few municipalities have recognized domestic partnerships. A few private companies have done the same. Employees of these municipalities and their lovers may be provided with some of the benefits, including insurance, usually provided only to married couples. If you work for a city government, inquire of a gay service organization to see if any benefits are provided for your lover.

Should you have to leave your job because of illness, or because you've been laid off, a federal law protects your insurance. It's called COBRA, and it covers all private companies with twenty or more employees. Under this law, and regardless of your medical condition, you can continue your group coverage, paying the group rate, for a period of eighteen months. If you stopped working because you are legally disabled (for example, if you have been diagnosed with AIDS), your coverage continues for an additional eleven months, for a total of twenty-nine months.

The COBRA law even helps get around the waiting period for preexisting conditions. Let's say you leave one employer to work for another, but the medical insurance of the new employer has a waiting period of one year. You have the option of continuing the coverage you received through your old employer (which covers the previous medical condition) until the one-year waiting period is up. You then drop the old coverage.

In light of the HIV epidemic, there are a few facts you should know about life insurance. For instance, the company can claim fraud on your application for only a period of two years from the date you applied. Most policies pay for suicide after the policy has been in force for two years, but not before. Many gay men are surprised to learn that you can't necessarily name anyone you want as your beneficiary. This is due to the stuffy, prudish morality of insurance companies. (Unmarried straights can't name their lovers as beneficiaries, either.) Unless you want to pursue a civil-rights case, there's no point in arguing with them or they may refuse to insure you. The usual tactic is to name either a relative or your estate as your beneficiary, and then change the beneficiary (to a lover or a friend) once the policy is in force (see *Wills*). In many states group life insurance can be converted to an individual policy, regardless of your health.

Some entrepreneurs have recently offered to "buy" the life insurance of AIDS patients, but at a discount. They argue that this provides money at a time when it's needed. You should be very careful about "selling" your life insurance. Getting advice from a lawyer is crucial, because you might be required to pay taxes on the proceeds, and/or become ineligible for Medicaid or other forms of public assistance.

Finally, let's note that many state laws are changing in ways that help the consumer. It is no longer possible for an employer to fire an employee because he's HIV-positive or has AIDS. One can even appeal the rejection of a claim by an insurance company because they claim the treatment is "experimental" or too costly. Your employer benefit book will explain how to do this. What is important for us gay people is to demand our insurance rights as often and as vocally as possible. This is usually accomplished through pressure on state insurance departments and via state laws. Those who work to lobby for favorable insurance laws have made and continue to make some of the most important advances in gay rights.

JEALOUSY, ENVY, AND POSSESSIVENESS

"Jealousy, which wears a bandage over its eyes, is not merely powerless to discover anything in the darkness that enshrouds it, it is also one of those torments where the task must be incessantly repeated." So wrote Marcel Proust in *Remembrance of Things Past,* that three-thousand-page dissection of this most destructive of all passions, jealousy: the compulsion that never discovers the truth and that can never be brought to a conclusion.

Jealousy is as rampant among homosexuals as among heterosexuals. Indeed, homosexuality provides so many more opportunities for quick, concealed sexual adventures that it is, if anything, a worse torture for the jealous man. If the nineteenth-century playwrights of bedroom farce had written about homosexuals the complications would have become still more riotous and confusing.

Jealousy is such an overwhelming emotion that it seems to the person afflicted by it to be innate and ineradicable. Despite this conviction, it is a learned emotion, often culturally inculcated, that exists far more often and with greater vehemence in some societies than in others. Since it is a learned response, it can also be unlearned.

The first step toward unlearning jealousy is recognizing the other feelings it probably conceals. Often jealousy is predicated on the belief that sex is the sole foundation of love. The jealous lover feels that his only hold over his partner is erotic and that once that physical grip is broken the lover will leave. In other words, *jealousy is a mask for the fear of abandonment.*

In other cases, jealousy is a projection of one's guilt about one's own peccadilloes. A man has sex on the sly with dozens of tricks, but each time he "cheats" he redoubles his interrogations and suspicions of his lover. He cannot face concealing his own adventures; the philandering is something he attributes to his lover, who may in fact be quite faithful.

Sometimes jealousy is a carryover from a heterosexual culture that places great emphasis on feminine chastity. A gay man from a Mediterranean or Latin family, for instance, may be as jealous of his lover as the straight men in his family are of their wives. Jealousy, in short, is only one aspect of an entire macho complex wherein his role is always that of the male, his lover's that of the female. A homosexual from such a background may be especially vehement because he feels guilty about being gay and attempts to prove his "masculinity," which he perceives as being diminished by his homosexuality.

In some cases jealousy is a smokescreen for envy. Bob says that he is jealous when his lover has sex with other people, but actually he wishes he could get tricks as fabulous as those Tom lands. If Bob were really honest with himself, he'd admit he's not plagued by jealousy over infidelity, but rather by his envy of Tom's successes. If Bob felt that he could attract men as easily as Tom, Bob would give up the pretense of being the jealous lover. Bob, though he doesn't acknowledge it, is in secret competition with Tom over sexual desirability and fears he may come in a poor second. Unfortunately, his low self-regard keeps this mental process unconscious to him, which guarantees constant bickering (if not outright abuse), and usually results in a broken relationship.

Many forms of jealousy are built upon possessiveness. A man believes and acts on the belief that his lover is his property, something he owns, and every time the lover has sex (or merely flirts) with outsiders the jealous man feels that his private estate has been plundered.

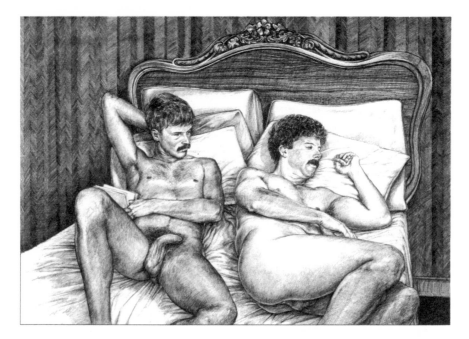

In virtually all cases, the immediate problem that brings on the rage felt by so many jealous men is a sudden, strongly perceived lack of self-worth. Jealousy is therefore not *between* two people, much as that would seem to be its field; it is completely self-generated. Indeed, jealousy is selfishness at its most extreme.

If you suffer from jealousy and wish to overcome it, you must first begin by admitting it's an emotion unworthy of you, one that is spoiling this affair and may well ruin all others in the future. As long as you hold on to the conviction that your jealousy is normal and justified, you will never beat it. Second, stop quizzing your lover and attempting to catch him out in lies and phony alibis. Avoid the temptation to read his diary, letters, or phone bills. Every time the fever attacks you, forget your lover's actions and examine your own emotions. What feelings lie under this frenzy? Guilt about homosexuality? Guilt about your own tricking? Envy? Uncertainty about whether your partner really loves you? If you are able to locate the deeper disturbance beneath jealousy, articulate it to your lover.

In many couples only one partner expresses jealousy, though both members contribute to its dynamics. If you and your lover are caught in the coils of jealousy, you should analyze your motives and actions. Sometimes one lover will feed the other's jealousy to keep him endlessly in suspense—and completely fascinated. Nothing is quite so binding as jealousy, at least if it's kept under control—the jealous lover never thinks of anything except his partner. If your relationship is held together by jealousy, you and your lover need to ask yourselves if you really need this interdependence and constant, subtle anguish to stay with each other.

J. O. BUDDIES

Jerk-off buddies are partners in fantasy. They talk dirty; they wear provocative costumes such as jockstraps, leather jackets, and chaps; and while they keep up a sex rap, they masturbate themselves and occasionally each other (see *Dirty Talk; Masturbation and Fantasy*). Some J.O. buddies operate long-distance, jerking off while talking on the phone. They describe themselves in erotic detail, talk about their cocks and sexual desires, and fantasize having sex together (see *Phone Sex*).

Still other J.O. buddies exchange letters, photographs, or audiotapes and videos of themselves. Sometimes they send each other their semen-stained underwear.

Jerking off with someone else is the preferred, sometimes the only, sexual outlet for some men (see *Computer Sex; J.O. Clubs; Phone Sex*). For others, it may be a form of foreplay or an exciting alternative to the more usual repertoire.

The fun of jerking off together is that you can live out fantasy scenes that would be either impossible or difficult to create in reality. (You don't really want to give up your job at the telephone company to become a cowboy). Some men get off on masochistic or sadistic fantasies but find the actuality of S/M gruesome; a J.O. buddy may be the perfect solution for them. Still others first got turned on by jerking off with a friend when they were younger, and this form of sex recalls for them their steamy, spermy youth.

The only drawback to jerking off as a dominant sexual habit is that it can become a substitute for the greater intimacy of lovemaking. Still, jerking off with a friend is a way of connecting with another man but maintaining distance, which probably explains its new prominence in this age of HIV Disease. Now you can be excited, get off sexually, and still enjoy completely safe sex.

J. O. CLUBS

J.O. clubs existed before the HIV crisis made safe sex absolutely necessary, but have become far more popular recently. Such clubs originated during the seventies, and were an outgrowth of private parties organized by gay guys who were into masturbation. They invited

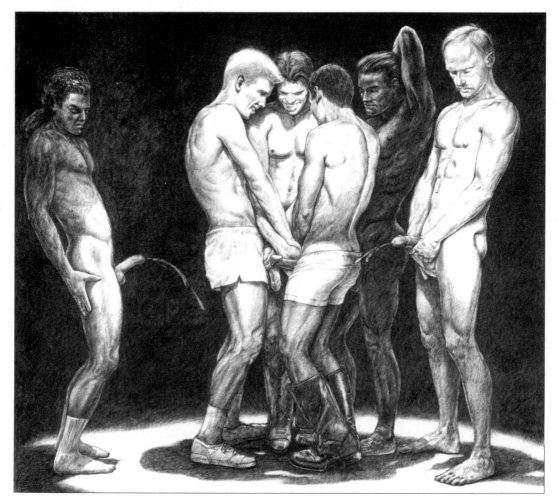

others who shared this interest to orgies where no sucking or fucking took place, only kissing, caressing, and jerking off (see *Orgies*). The group expanded, was named the Jacks (i.e., "those who jack off") and attracted not only exhibitionists and men with large penises (especially members of the Eight-Plus Club) but also those attracted to them. J.O. clubs soon became so crowded they had to move their biweekly parties to large loft spaces, and then to dance clubs during their "off" nights.

What makes J.O. clubs different from back rooms (which continue to exist, though in much-reduced numbers) is that penetration is forbidden. One member of Jacks says of the club that it is for "cocksmen and cock-worshipers" only. He explains that any penetration "hides" the cock. At J.O. clubs, it makes no difference whether you are fully dressed, partly dressed, or nude; tall, short, fat, thin, beautiful, or unattractive: If you have a large, or fat, or extra-long, or unusual cock, you will be popular. Also desired are men who come many times per night, or excite others while they're jerking off.

A J.O. club is usually dimly lit, with pulsating music; it's a whirlpool of sounds, smells, and sensations. Instead of lying on beds, couches, or banquettes, everyone stands, and moves from one knot of activity to another and from one group to another. Hand towels and lubricants are made available upon entering, and in some cases, there is a lounge where no sex is taking place and where refreshments are served.

J.O. clubs have lately been evolving into sex clubs where unsafe sex is making a reappearance. You should be extra careful in these kinds of clubs. Consider this: The men you're having sex with may have already had sex with numerous other men during the night. STDs and HIV are among the uninvited guests. (See *Sex Clubs*.)

KISSING

A kiss is both a romantic symbol and an erotic act, and this dual nature makes kisses deliciously ambiguous. The lips are among the most sensitive parts of the body, rivaled only by the fingertips and palms. The mouth is the baby's first organ of pleasure, and throughout adult life a person continues to suck, taste, lick, chew, and swallow as ways of deriving enjoyment.

A sexy kiss is not a chaste peck but a deep and varied exploration, not just of your partner's mouth but of his whole body. When you kiss, your mouth should be wet; a dry mouth is not very appealing. Run your tongue over the sensitive surface of his gums, between the teeth and upper lip. Reach with your tongue to the top of his mouth and dart the tip over those delicate membranes—penetration of his mouth with your tongue is the classic and highly erotic French, or soul, kiss. Suck his tongue; nibble his lower lip; lick his nostrils; smear a kiss down his neck to that hollow just above

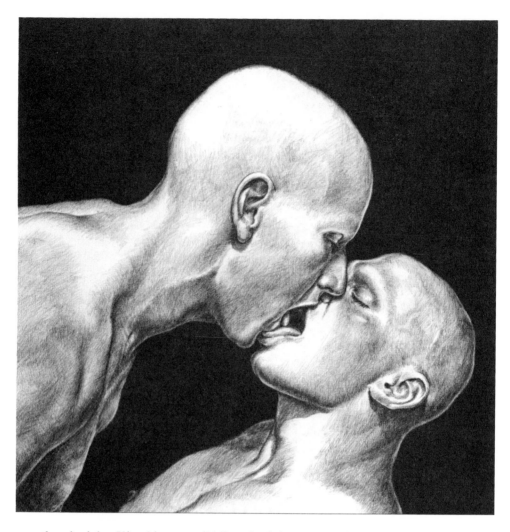

the clavicle. Kiss his ear, nibbling the lobe or scouring the whole interior with your tongue; then draw back and exhale warm breath onto the ear.

Some men, of course, resist kissing. This resistance is often a last hold-out against a full commitment to homosexuality ("Cowboys don't kiss"). Hustlers who think of themselves as straight don't kiss; soldiers or sailors who offer themselves as "straight" trade refuse to kiss. When young adolescent boys first start fooling around with each other, they also often draw the line at kissing. As long as their lips never meet, they can rationalize that what they're doing (and it can be anything from sixty-nining to what was once called cornholing) is not homosexual, but just "getting their rocks off." Kissing is the heart of romance. In sex between men the final pledge of intimacy is offered not by the degree of ardor or penetration or abandon during sex but by the depth and the tenderness of a kiss.

Of course, kisses needn't be tender. They can be cool and contemplative or rough and aggressive. The mouth is not only for sucking and licking but also for biting (see *Nibbling and Biting*). Your partner may not like you to be rough, so ask him.

Whether rough or gentle, kissing is an integral part of the entire experience of making love. Most men like to get fucked lying on their backs precisely so that they can kiss during sex. Before or after fucking, a kiss on the lips merges into a pilgrimage over your partner's body—the hot erogenous zones of the nipples, the toes and fingers, the palms of the hands, or the hollows of the armpits. Your lover will tell you where he likes to be kissed; a trick probably will not, but you can usually get a good idea of what he wants done by noticing and imitating what he does to you.

Just how important kissing is in truly gratifying sex can be gauged by a popular slang complaint about being unsatisfied: "Fucked without a kiss!"

LETTING GO

In Orwell's novel *Nineteen Eighty-four,* O'Brien asks, "What is the worst thing in the world?" For most of us it is feeling unloved and abandoned. These are the primary feelings experienced when a love relationship ends. Sometimes the lovers have been quarreling for years. For other couples, months or years of silent distance abruptly end as one partner announces, to the astonishment of the other, that their relationship is over. No matter how long the relationship has lasted, and no matter how the end comes about, termination is painful for both parties—sometimes devastating to one; sometimes devastating to both.

What is worse, some men can't let go of the past. They tenaciously hold on to the conviction that "he still loves me," in the face of overwhelming evidence to the contrary. Invariably, the holder-on is obsessed with finding evidence that his former lover still loves him. These indications turn out to be flagrant distortions. The personality and character of the beloved are transformed into something approaching saintliness. Unkind acts are reinterpreted as benevolent; even abuse can be reinterpreted as love (see *Domestic Violence*). This is *obsessive love,* and its effects are harmful all the time.

Relationships do not always work out (see *Couples*). It may not be either's fault. Two men may have gotten together because of sexual compatibility, mistaking that for love. Over time, one or both may lose interest, or one changes in important ways while the other doesn't. Even so, once a breakup occurs, both are likely to feel depressed (see *Depression*).

The obsessed man continues to pursue his lost love, while friends familiar with the situation look on with amazement. The beloved, meanwhile, may be furious and resentful over being hounded. It does no good to tell someone, "It's over," if he simply does not or cannot believe it. For him, reconciling himself to such rejection would be equivalent to admitting he's no more than a little boy lost in the forest.

There are no cures for men who are obsessed over a former lover, or over unrequited love. Psychologists have learned that these are the most obdurate obsessions, and the most difficult to relieve in psychotherapy. This is because the obsessed lover rejects much of the world and focuses only on the beloved. The obsession is dispelled only when the man opens his life again to meeting new people. Friends can be helpful in this process.

The beloved can make things better or worse, depending upon how he ended the relationship and on his subsequent behavior. If you are ending a love relationship, tell your lover why. Don't leave it to his imagination. Make your complaints as specific as possible. If you're willing, try couples therapy, but don't do so if you know in your heart you want to be free of him. Otherwise you will only breed further resentment. Be as clear as you can about what further contact you want with him. Avoid ambiguous statements, since they cause misperceptions. If you don't want any contact with him in the future, come out and say so. Make it clear that you won't allow friends to be used as intermediaries.

The problem of unrequited love is similar but not the same. Most of us have fallen madly in love with someone who either never knew of our passion or who, if he did, showed no romantic interest in return. Most of us get over it in time, but some men pursue the love object and become furiously jealous at the success of competitors (see *Jealousy, Envy, and Possessiveness*). A few men become so angry that they interfere in the life of the beloved. Naturally, the beloved sees only the insanity of it all: His life is being intruded upon by a madman.

If you are a man being hounded by an obsessed or unrequited lover, here's what you should do to make it clear that you have no interest in him whatsoever. State without the slightest ambiguity that you are not interested. Make it clear that you will not meet or talk to him, in person or over the phone. Send back cards and presents mailed or delivered to you. Then inform all mutual friends not to transmit any information between you.

Last, cross your fingers and hope that all this works.

Grieving over the death of a lover or close friend is a particularly painful part of the process of letting go. HIV Disease has produced a legion of young widowers who need to grieve for their losses while continuing to function effectively in the world. Some survivors have a terrible time of it; they suffer deep, long-lasting depression. A few accuse themselves of not doing enough and end up guilt-ridden. It's also common for the survivor to feel abandoned by his dead lover, and resentful toward him. Some others refuse to throw out or give away any of the dead man's possessions. Finally, some men launch themselves into frequent sexual encounters. All these are ways to cover up the pain.

If you have trouble letting go, see a therapist who will help you with the process. Friends can help to a certain extent, but sometimes feel inadequate to the task. Support groups for survivors may suggest particular techniques for accepting the loss.

It's very common for survivors to talk to the dead lover. If you do this, don't stop. Talk to him and tell him how you feel, what life is like without him. Express whatever feelings well up in you, both the loving and the angry ones. And cry—or break something. Take some minor possession of his (nothing with emotional significance) and, while throwing it out, tell him you're doing so. Tell him (and yourself) that that physical object has nothing to do with your love for him. Another day, throw out or give away another possession. One day, when you're ready, you'll dispose of most of his belongings, but keep items that remind you of the good times. But disposing of possessions is the easy part. More difficult is not only accepting his death, but recognizing that a part of you has also died.

LIVING WILLS

The living will is a relatively new legal instrument. About thirty-five states permit one to make a living will, which clarifies your wishes regarding medical treatment if, because of a serious accident or profound illness, you are unable to make such decisions for yourself. As a rule, what is at stake here is control of your body, its upkeep and maintenance, when you are not in a position to make your wishes known. The living will stipulates which, if any, life-sustaining mechanisms you want used to prolong your life, and for how long. Some people feel that these treatments, such as breathing machines, liquid nutrition, and cardiac resuscitation, only serve to draw out the agonies of death. They also feel that such extended dying periods only increase the pain of lovers and family members.

As several of the specific illnesses suffered by those in the latter stages of AIDS can lead to coma or mental disorganization, those with the disease often make out living wills.

Lawyers suggest that you give someone a *medical power of attorney* to make these decisions. You can designate anyone you want. New York State has a health-care proxy law that allows you to declare your health-care decisions and name a surrogate to make dispositions on your behalf. This is not possible in many other states. One may also name a conservator, who is empowered to make *any* decision in your name—medical, financial, or business. The nomination of a conservator is obviously the most powerful protection you have, assuming that the conservator is one you trust and who makes wise decisions. These alternatives should be discussed with your attorney, preferably one who understands the social and legal problems of gay people.

You shouldn't keep a living will a secret. Copies of it should go to everyone who has an interest in it. This includes your family, your lover, your physicians, and your hospital. But it isn't enough to give them copies;

you also need to speak to each in person, so that they have a clear idea of your intentions. Be careful about choosing a hospital run under the auspices of a religious group. Some will refuse to curtail treatment no matter what legal documents are brought to bear. Others seem to have no standard guidelines for abiding by living wills; they decide on a case-by-case basis. Under these circumstances you or your caretaker may be forced into the position of taking the hospital to court for your right to die.

Finally, don't confuse a living will with a will. You can think of both as documents that speak for you, but a living will speaks for you only until your death. After that, only a will speaks for you (see *Insurance; Wills*).

LONELINESS

Feeling alone is frightening and depressing. No matter how much money or status a man may have, no matter how many friends and tricks he can point to, he may still be besieged by an intolerable sense of alienation. Even a man with a devoted lover may experience profound isolation.

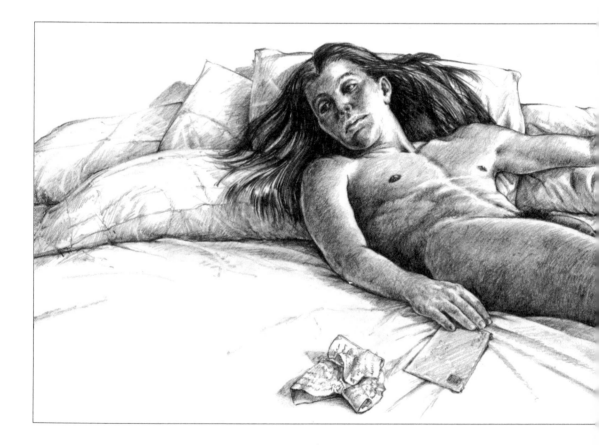

There are three kinds of loneliness—two that must be accepted, and a third that can be fought. First is the loneliness caused by the death of a very close friend, a lover, or a member of one's family. The resulting sadness is always appropriate because the loss is real, not symbolic (see *Depression; Letting Go*). A second isolation that must be accepted is "cosmic" loneliness. Often an individual in his thirties or forties, who has buried the ghosts of his past, freed himself from any neurotic aspects of his relationships with his parents, his boss, and his lover, and achieved a clear-eyed view of himself—often this person will suddenly be hit hard by the full force of cosmic loneliness, what William James called vastation in *The Varieties of Religious Experience:* the adult recognition that we are born alone and will die alone, and that many of our private experiences will never be successfully shared with other people. There's nothing to be done about that.

But the third kind of loneliness can be combated. Though we don't think of it this way, the usual kind of aching loneliness is something we ourselves have created. This loneliness is our rejection of other people, our refusal to let them become a significant part of our lives. A lonely man might say, even when he is surrounded by thousands of other gays, that he cannot relate to any of them. He will claim that all they want is sex, not intimacy,

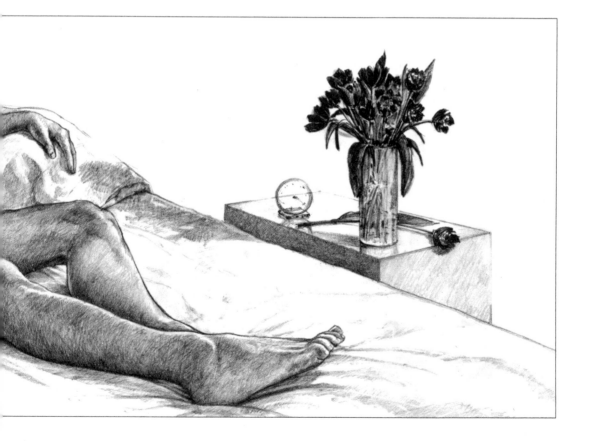

whereas it is he who demands sex and fears affection. In order to keep intact his conviction that no one is loving, the lonely man will seek unloving men. He may marry and live a double life, and then curse his inability to find male love because he is imprisoned by his marriage, a situation of his own making.

One of the most common forms of loneliness among gay men, even in these days of HIV infection, afflicts those who consciously desire to have nothing but anonymous, quick sex. Having contrived a world of quick sex for themselves, they then complain that quick sex is all that gay men ever want. Since they lack respect for themselves, they show an equal disrespect for their sex partners by not respecting safe sex guidelines and therefore endangering both lives. (Of course there are also gay men who have nothing but anonymous sex, enjoy it, and don't complain about it.)

If you are caught in a trap of loneliness of your own devising, then you ought to consider changing your habits. Plan purely social times with your friends, rather than going out cruising. Love and friendship are not airtight compartments; if you can achieve intimacy with a friend, you may also be preparing yourself for eventual closeness with a lover. Meet new people in new places, or approach new people in the old places in a different way. Perhaps you shouldn't jump into bed with someone you meet at the gym; ask him out for dinner or a movie, talk to him, court him. If trying out new approaches frightens you, no matter. Better to feel anxious but change than to remain safely in a neurotic pattern that one poet has characterized as "old, inadequate and flourishing."

LUBRICANTS

Essential for fucking, often a real help when masturbating yourself, fun for a "slip and slide" jerk-off session with someone else, lubricants come in many varieties. Some are expensive, flavored, scented, and marketed under coy or erotic names. Others are cheaper, more practical, and as close as your grocery shelf or drugstore. Take the water-soluble lubricants, such as K-Y, a favorite among gays as it is easily washed off bodies and sheets. The only trouble with water-soluble lubricants is that they can dry out in mid-ecstasy. Petroleum jelly (Vaseline) and vegetable shortening are cheap and good bets, since they stay greasy for hours, but they are not water-soluble, and therefore should *never* be used with latex condoms because they degrade the latex. Crisco is the favorite of serious fisters (see *Fisting*).

The newest lubricants contain spermicides (sperm killers), which kill many of the bacterial agents that cause disease (see *Sexually Transmitted Diseases*). These new "safer" lubricants come in all sorts of packages, from plastic jars to pocket-sized tubes, and they contain water-soluble nonoxynol-9, which kills the HIV virus. One such lubricant is called ForPlay. Many safe lubricants come in the package with condoms, making them especially handy for AIDS prevention.

MARRIED MEN

For centuries gays have married to perpetuate their names, or to achieve respectability in business and in the community. Homosexuality was ''the love that dares not speak its name'' for so long that marriage seemed necessary to create a family. Many men still marry for these same reasons, and lead a double life.

But the pattern is changing. Some men divulge their homosexuality to their wives so as to enrich the marriage and make it more honest. Such confessions are usually painful to make and painful to hear. If resentment, recrimination, and bitterness overwhelm the couple, the marriage will end in divorce.

Why do gay men marry? There are three reasons. First, some gay men arrive at adulthood already having an intimate and erotic relationship with a woman. A surprising number of ''childhood sweethearts'' fit this pattern. Although these men sleep with their wives with pleasure (or not, as the case may be), they're not sexually interested in other women. For extramarital

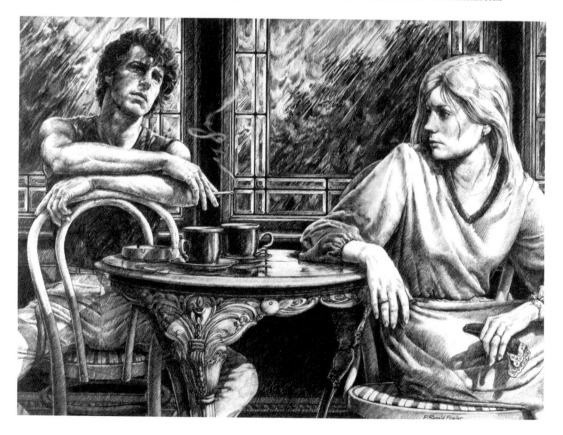

adventures, they turn to men. Some of these men have married to fulfill their longing for children; childlessness can be a significant frustration in gay life.

A second group is gay men who marry to please their parents and their social network.

Third, some men in therapy claim they're pleasing their straight therapists. Marriage often brings high praise from straight therapists, who generally regard the marriage as a sign the patient has been successfully treated. The "success" is an illusion on both parts. The straight therapist who urges his gay male patient to marry is particularly reprehensible and the source of a great deal of woe. The marriage is also cruel to the wife who doesn't know she's a "cure" rather than the object of love. With or without therapists, some gay men marry to "cure themselves" of their homosexuality.

All these men know they're gay: They've had gay sex before and they understand perfectly well that they'll continue to have it after marriage. They make time for gay sex by lying to their wives, but as with all deceptions they experience anxiety and guilt.

Married gay men face daunting problems, which are especially acute for those who conceal their homosexuality. They worry about transmitting disease to their wives. Smart husbands confine their gay sex to one or two known men.

One solution for the married gay man is to have an affair with another married man. Each understands the limitations of the relationship. If their wives or their children become friends, the men can be together on trips, during vacations, and at parties.

Problems may develop if a married gay man falls in love with someone single. The gay single pesters his married lover for more time together—always difficult to arrange. Or the married man may decide to leave his wife. This is such a big step that it can severely test, and often end, the gay relationship. For the single gay man, the dangers of being in love with a married man should be obvious. All the *Back Street* movies ever made suddenly seem appallingly real instead of cheaply sentimental, and nothing in the world will compensate for him being with *her* when you want him with you.

Probably the best combination is the horny, younger, married gay man with the older, career-driven or otherwise strongly involved single gay man. They should most appreciate each other's delimited time, sexual involvement, and company—without the heartaches and the messy emotional house cleaning afterward.

Today, married men can join support groups with other married men. These groups are usually anonymous; they're organized by gay community centers throughout the country.

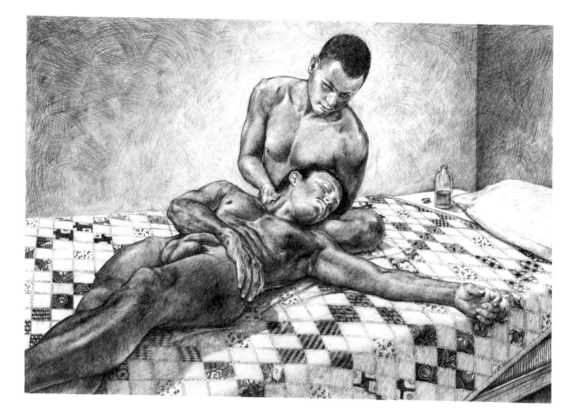

MASSAGE

There are two basic kinds of massage. One is primarily intended to reduce muscle tension and might be administered by a masseur at the gym or might be recommended by a doctor to a patient who had, say, a lower back problem.

The other kind, our concern here, is an explicit attempt to bring sensual pleasure to the person being massaged.

The sensuous massage gives people permission to accept pleasure. In ordinary sexual situations, many people are uptight about receiving pleasure; they can give it, but they have trouble accepting it (see *Pleasure Trap*). When a person is receiving massage, however, accepting pleasure becomes a specific and conscious *assignment*. A sex therapist will handle such patients very firmly, ordering them to lie passively on a bed and soak up the sensations offered. The therapist, in other words, has taken charge of the situation and assumed responsibility for whatever happens. Pleasure-resistant people are finally able to relax and submit to the doctor's orders. This clinical arrangement can also be adapted to informal massage sessions between friends, lovers, or fuck buddies.

After someone has learned to relax, he should indicate when something feels good and when it doesn't (''More light stroking over there, please'').

People need to ask for what feels good. By learning to ask during a massage, they prepare to make their desires known to their sexual partners.

Massage reduces anxiety and tension not only because it turns the acceptance of pleasure into an assignment, but also, oddly enough, because it explicitly excludes sexual activity. The culprit it thus avoids is performance anxiety—the dread that you won't function adequately during sex—a fear that can become entrenched and self-perpetuating after repeated failure. Sensual massage is a way of overcoming performance anxiety by bringing two people into physical contact under a ban against sex. If you know that no matter how aroused you become you will not be permitted to have sex, your performance anxiety will gradually ebb away.

There are several types of sensual massage, described in ascending order, up to the most arousing. You should both be naked while doing all types of massage.

The first calls for the two participants to take turns rubbing each other. The man giving the massage moves with light, caressing strokes from the head and face down to the feet and toes. You might want to use a soft powder to smooth out your hands.

At every point, the person receiving the massage gives instructions for more or less pressure on this or that part of the body. The erogenous zones are scrupulously avoided; the masseur does not stroke the nipples, balls, cock, or anus. If the man being stroked becomes sexually aroused he should not be allowed to shift into sex play. After the first man has been massaged, they switch places.

The second type, the genital massage, permits the masseur to rub the erogenous zones, but he must stroke the genitals in exactly the same way he strokes other parts of the body. The masseur should not linger more over the cock, say, than the thighs or arms, and he should by no means masturbate his partner. The object is not to induce an erection or to bring about climax but to provide pleasure, pure and simple. Both men should take note of their erotic fantasies.

Afterward, both participants compare notes. Some men's inhibitions about having fantasies and communicating them interfere with a rich, satisfying sex life. By becoming aware of and reporting their fantasies (even the most fleeting erotic thoughts) during massage, they can begin to overcome their reticence.

After the participants have tried out light, sensual massage and the somewhat more arousing genital massage, they might move on to direct sexual massage. Sexual massage may be the prelude to more intense sexual activity. The couple can use oils and powders; they can stroke each other not only with hands but also with mouth, lips, tongue, vibrators, dildos, or whatever suits their fancy. This form of massage need not be as gentle as the other two; it can get as rough as they like. The participants may take turns or rub each other simultaneously, or combine massage with sucking, fucking, and other sexual acts.

MASTURBATION
AND FANTASY

T he ancient Egyptians believed that the Nile rose each year because of the continual masturbation of the god Osiris, and that all living things were created by his semen. It's unfortunate that this positive view of masturbation didn't survive into the Judeo-Christian era.

For centuries, masturbation has been condemned and persecuted in Western society, first by religious authorities and then by those modern watchdogs of morality, the medical profession. In the eighteenth century, the moral condemnation of masturbation was reinterpreted as a medical issue: Masturbation became an illness as well as a sin. A widely influential French physician, Tissot, said masturbation destroyed the nervous system, resulting in madness.

In 1834 Dr. Sylvester Graham wrote that the loss of semen during sex was injurious to health (a popular idea at the time); men, Graham believed, should not have intercourse more than twelve times a year. Masturbation was especially pernicious. To reduce sexual cravings, Graham advised mild foods to decrease sexual appetites. The graham cracker was the result! In 1884, this curious connection between food and sex appeared in another guise. Dr. John Harvey Kellogg created cornflakes to curtail children's inclinations toward masturbation. Kellogg, a bit of a flake himself, wrote: "The *use* of the reproductive function is perhaps the highest physical act of which man is capable; its *abuse* is certainly one of the most grievous outrages against nature which it is possible for him to perpetrate."

From this period on, parents told children that awful things would happen if they touched their genitals: Hair would grow on the palms of their hands, or their brains would become "soft." Since even "good" children might masturbate in their sleep, some fearful parents enclosed children's arms in cardboard cuffs.

Still, the warnings were ignored, and children went on playing with their genitals. The protests (somewhat hysterical) continued. William Acton, a prominent physician, wrote: "There is now in Pennsylvania—it seems unnecessary to name the place—a man thirty-five years old, with the infirmities of 'three score and ten.' Yet his premature old age, his bending and tottering form, wrinkled face, and hoary head, might be traced to solitary and social *licentiousness*."

Between 1856 and 1919 the U.S. Patent Office granted patents for forty-nine antimasturbation devices. Thirty-five were for horses and fourteen for humans. The human devices, made for boys, consisted of either sharp points turned inward to jab the boy's penis should he get an erection, or an electrical system to deliver shocks. We don't know how many of these devices were actually used, or what effect they had on the children.

Although masturbation in men was repeatedly denounced, female masturbation was opposed with even greater ferocity. Women who masturbated were regarded by the nineteenth-century medical profession as manifesting dangerously masculine appetites. Starting in 1858, some women were subjected to clitoridectomy, which effectively removed all possibility of clitoral pleasure; this operation continued as a treatment for female masturbators until 1937, even though it had been discredited by the medical profession a half century earlier.

In the twentieth century, masturbation was rediagnosed by psychiatrists as a sexual perversion. Though they did not go so far as to say masturbation would lead to insanity, they did suggest it led to "abnormal" sexual development and, some feared, homosexuality—which some psychiatrists *did* believe was a form of insanity. Until 1968, masturbation remained listed as a mental disorder in the American Psychiatric Association's *Diagnostic and Statistical Manual*. Even today, many psychiatrists say that masturbation is not in itself a disorder—unless practiced too much. In other words, it's accepted as a substitute for heterosexual intercourse when that is unavailable, but anyone who chooses to masturbate rather than have sex is regarded as infantile or disturbed. (Read *Homosexuality and American Psychiatry: The Politics of Diagnosis* by Ronald Bayer.)

The goal of all this diagnosis was to create internalized feelings of guilt about masturbatory behavior, thereby marshaling people to police their own thoughts and actions. "No self-indulgence," says the superego (the Jiminy Cricket sitting on one's shoulder), "or I will punish you by making you feel like shit" (see *Guilt*). Men who don't start masturbating until their twenties have learned that lesson particularly well, but few can claim to have grown up in our sexually repressed society without any hang-ups about jerking off.

A view that seems to us much more rational, productive, and realistic is that masturbation is not just a substitute to be tolerated, but a necessary requirement for proper psychosexual development. Only if boys and girls are permitted to masturbate freely and shamelessly will they be able to chart the contours of their own sexual desires. The physical reactions and imaginative ideation produced during masturbation allow the individual to define his or her sexual tastes and build confidence. The enjoyment derived from masturbation promotes greater acceptance of physical pleasure in general and of one's own body in particular.

A gay man incapable of a little fantasizing during sex is probably not very passionate. More than likely, he sticks to a rigid sequence of acts and is frightened and bewildered by the extent of other people's sexual inventiveness. Fantasies, therefore, are highly desirable, and masturbation is the best classroom for developing the fantasy faculty.

One helpful teaching aid is pornography. Some gay men are turned on by photos, others by sexy, stylized drawings, still others by stories or videotapes (see *Pornography*). Discover which media and styles excite you: Naked or clothed figures? Alone or engaged in sex with others? Which details excite you? Which sexual practices do you prefer to look at? Of

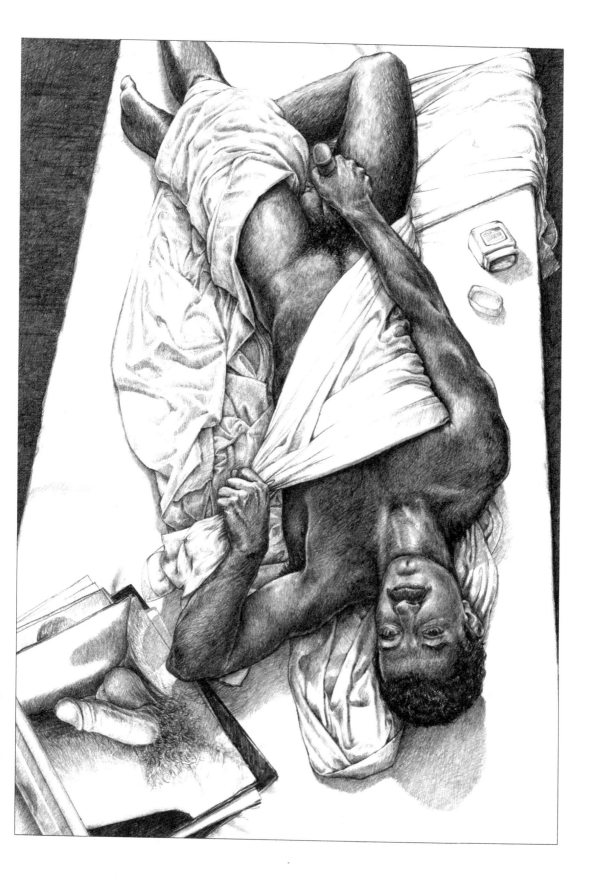

course, some men prefer to use their imagination to relive a stimulating episode or summon up an exciting person from their own past. Perhaps they saw some really sexy guy walking up the street this morning, or had a really hot sex scene with someone last week, or even just liked looking at the beautiful body of a friend at the beach. It's not unusual for vigorous and horny men to vividly recall and jerk off less than an hour following a particularly exciting sexual encounter.

Pick a quiet time and take the pornography you've selected to bed with you. Create a soothing environment, with low lights and music or whatever relaxes you. Look through the pictures and choose one that turns you on. Concentrate on that picture and invent a story about it, one that also involves you. As your cock starts to get hard, continue the fantasy and begin to masturbate. If you've never used a lubricant, try one, such as K-Y, baby lotion, or Vaseline—everyone has his favorite (see *Lubricants*). Be sure to keep up the fantasy until you reach a climax. Your stories may become as elaborate and as kinky as you like.

If you practice fantasizing while masturbating for several days, you can attempt to transfer sexual fantasizing to encounters with other men. Some partners, you'll discover, are particularly adept at collaborating in your fantasies. They talk during sex, expanding on the things you say and do, and will even act out quite elaborate scenes involving costumes, fetishes, and let's-pretend situations (army barracks, a locker room, the men's room on an airplane, and so on).

Jerking off with a partner has become the highlight of some men's sexual lives (see *J.O. Buddies; J.O. Clubs*). Still, men who feel guilty about jerking off ask, "Am I doing it too much?" You'll know you are when your body tells you. The skin on your cock shaft or glans will become chafed, or your dick may ache from being handled too much. Frequency of masturbation, like frequency of sex in general, is a measure of libido, boredom, anxiety, and a number of other factors, none of which is harmful. There can be one problem, however.

Sometimes, a man will so finely tune his masturbatory technique that no one else can get him off. A partner often feels inadequate when that happens. One way of dealing with the situation is to cup your hand over your partner's hand and use his hand to jerk yourself off. That will show him how you like it done.

Having said all this, we should point out that the function of masturbatory fantasies is not simply to rehearse for play-acting with sexual partners. Many men like to keep their masturbatory fantasies private, and the things they conjure up during masturbation they would never do with anyone else. The links between fantasy and reality are subtle and complex, so sharing your fantasy with another person might not suit you at all. Of course, if your lover is understanding, he will recognize that the roles you play in bed do not need to be carried into the rest of your lives. But if you want to keep your fantasies private, fine; their only function is to redirect your focus from the mechanics of sexuality to its creative spirit and to shift your attention from meeting someone else's expectations to fulfilling your own.

Finally, we end this essay with a quote from another physician, Dr. Thomas Cogan, who in 1589 wrote:

> The commodities which come by moderate evacuation thereof [that is, of semen] are great. For it procureth appetite to meat and helpeth concoction; it maketh the body more light and nimble, it openeth the pores and conduits, and purgeth phlegm; it quickeneth the mind, stirreth up the wit, reneweth the sense, driveth away sadness, madness, anger, melancholy, fury.

What modern writer could have said it better?

MIRRORS

Not the mirrors you look into while shaving or to check the crease of your trousers. Mirrors used in sex can be any size and shape, and can be placed anywhere. One mirror or several, placed around the bed or staring down from the ceiling, can double your pleasure. To the joy

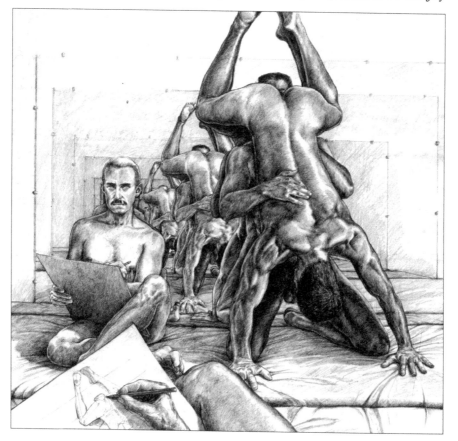

of direct sexual involvement with your partner they add another pleasure, that of watching yourselves. You can pretend you're a porno star. Mirrors can show you intriguing new angles on yourself and your partner during what may have become boring positions and activities. They can turn a duo into an illusory foursome. The more mirrors you have, the more fully you can see details and the whole scene; no matter what position you choose, you'll otherwise miss an angle or two.

Some men have become such looking-glass addicts they've mirrored their bedrooms, their dressing rooms, their bathrooms. But others are afraid of being branded narcissists, and therefore avoid mirrors as though they cast evil spells. A bit more narcissism would make most men more secure about their bodies, especially when they check out exactly what each part looks like, from different perspectives, in varied positions, aroused or not.

MIXED HIV COUPLES

Coming inside your lover, or having him come inside of you, has always been one of the joys of gay sex. These pleasures must now be curtailed, replaced by safe sex practices, especially when one lover is HIV-positive and the other HIV-negative (see *Safe Sex*). Simple, yet practical measures can ensure that the virus isn't transmitted from one to the other. These include keeping toothbrushes and razors separate (perhaps by color-coding?), and not kissing after flossing one's teeth. While such practical measures are easily undertaken, it's the emotional upheaval of HIV that most threatens the relationship between lovers.

It's a shock to learn that one is HIV-positive (see *Body Positive*). Some men are capable of ignoring the implications of such a diagnosis, and carry on with their lives and their lovers much as they did before. Most men, however, are thrown into turmoil and need time to come to terms with the consequences of this new knowledge. The couple is threatened by the overwhelming fear of illness and death. There is also another terrible fear: that the HIV-positive lover may transmit the virus to his HIV-negative lover. Many new infections have indeed been transmitted in this manner. Perhaps one member of the couple didn't know about his seropositive status, and inadvertently passed on the infection. Others, concealing their secret out of fear of abandonment, have risked exposing the other partner. Finally, the seropositive person is terrified that he will be abandoned by his lover at the very time he needs him most. The HIV-positive person isn't likely to mention this fear to his lover, because he recognizes its irrationality.

Guilt is another ingredient in this emotional stew. The seropositive man may feel guilty about his former sexual behavior. The seronegative partner may feel guilty not for what he's done, but rather for what he feels. His first reaction may be panic (though he's not likely to show it). "I want out of here," he may say to himself, "but I'm trapped." He's frightened that he may become infected, yet he feels that he can never leave the relationship. The healthy lover, who is frightened for himself, often compensates by taking charge of his infected lover's life, treating him as if he's physically and mentally crippled. This is likely to drive both men crazy.

Love in a relationship means many things. One is the freedom to ventilate feelings and reveal vulnerabilities that surface when danger threatens. The combination of guilt, depression, abandonment, and resentment can only be handled when lovers talk about these feelings truthfully. It's a scary but necessary process. It's also a good idea for both men to have support groups to help them with their feelings and to get advice from those in a similar situation. This is a time when friendship can be most valuable. Occasionally, a therapist may be called in to help the communication process.

Lovers usually agree about whom should be told about the diagnosis. Some seropositive men want to keep the information close to home and divulge it to very few, while others tell everyone. There are no rights or wrongs here. Occasionally, however, a seropositive man will ask his lover not to talk about it to anyone. This is unfair. The healthy lover needs to be able to express his fears.

What about sex? There is no reason to curtail it. But what often happens is that the uninfected lover starts to treat his partner like fragile porcelain, while the other lover still wants to have the same sort of sex as that they shared before the diagnosis. If he liked a rough fuck before, he doesn't want to be touched like a scared virgin now.

An HIV-positive man doesn't want to be treated like fine crystal outside the bedroom either. If you've always complained to him about some aspect of his behavior (say, not helping around the house), don't stop complaining now because of his diagnosis. Hard though it may be, don't show an exaggerated concern over every cough, groan, or pimple. And don't stare at him.

At some point you'll feel comfortable enough to talk about the future. You'll want to get your financial and health plans in order (see *Insurance; Living Wills; Wills*). Then get on with your life together.

MYTHIC BEGINNINGS

One tribe in New Guinea believes that homosexuality results from eating the meat of uncircumcised pigs. The Western world has invented other theories, no less imaginative, but none has been substantiated. For that matter, no scientist has ever explained how people end up heterosexual, a matter every bit as mysterious.

Theories about the origin of homosexuality can be divided into three categories: folk, physiological, and psychological. The most common folk theory holds that boys become gay if they are molested by experienced older homosexuals (this is called the recruitment theory). But childhood seduction has no demonstrable influence upon the later sexual preference of the child. The trauma of childhood sexual abuse may make the individual fearful of *all* sex later in life, but it will not influence his sexual orientation (see *Early Abuse*). The recruitment theory is in reality nothing more than a smokescreen, designed to hide the fact that most child molestation is heterosexual and occurs within the family.

A second folk theory based upon modeling holds that boys grow up to be gay if their fathers are weak and ineffectual. Such a theory equates homosexuality with inadequacy, a dubious identification. Moreover, it ignores the fact that more than half of marriages end in divorce and a substantial number of children grow up without a father in the house. There is not a shred of evidence that sexual orientation is influenced either by divorce (no matter how bitter) or by the absence of the father.

Still another folk theory holds that gay men are afraid of women. This idea is sometimes called the *vagina dentata* theory; it is based upon the notion that a gay man hates his mother, and transfers that hate to all other women. Needless to say, there is no better support for this folk theory than for the others, and it ignores the fact that many gay men have had, and will continue to have, satisfying sexual experiences with women.

The first person to propose a biological theory for the origin of homosexuality was the philosopher Aristotle. He wondered why some men liked to get fucked. In explanation, he suggested that such people had an extra nerve that ran to the rectum, which, he hypothesized, was stimulated during intercourse. Though ingenious, Aristotle's extra-nerve theory doesn't hold up anatomically.

A nineteenth-century French doctor, A. Tardieu, claimed that the active pederast had a slender, underdeveloped penis tapered like a dog's, and that those assuming the "passive" role in anal intercourse had smooth rectums. One wonders how anyone could come up with anything so preposterous.

A number of biological theories were proposed throughout the twentieth century to explain homosexuality. The simplest was genetic: Homosexuality is inherited. This is hotly debated.

The next biological theory was based upon hormone levels. Simple-minded psychologists and psychiatrists suggested that gay men had excessive female hormones (estrogens) circulating in their bodies, but were deficient in male hormones (androgens). After decades of research the theory was found to be completely in error. There are no demonstrable hormonal differences between persons with different sexual orientations.

The most recent biological theory holds that sexual orientation is determined in the brain of the fetus during the fourth to seventh month of pregnancy. Devotees of this prenatal theory suggest that the brain develops as either male or female. They say an "abnormality" may cause the male fetus's brain to develop into a female brain and that such a boy is destined to become an adult homosexual. Conversely, a male brain in a female is said to produce an adult lesbian.

The prenatal theory, like the others, has foundered on the rock of hard evidence. However, research in endocrinology may one day reveal the secret of sexual orientation. For the moment, biological explanations of homosexuality remain hotly contested. Recent anatomical studies have suggested differences between male and female brains, and between the brains of gay and straight men. How the data from anatomical studies will fit in with that from prenatal hormonal research remains to be seen.

There have been just as many psychological theories. The first (and the quaintest) we know of was suggested by a Persian physician a few hundred years ago. He wondered why so many Persian men preferred to have anal intercourse with young boys rather than vaginal intercourse with their wives. He believed that preference for vaginal or anal intercourse was determined by how a man learned to masturbate. He said that men were either "pounders" or "flippers." Pounders held their dicks very tightly and in adulthood preferred the tightness of a boy's asshole, while flippers held their dicks loosely and therefore enjoyed the wideness of a woman's vagina. While obviously incorrect about the origin of sexual orientation, the theory allows us a small window through which to view a past society that was more positive than our own about both masturbation and anal intercourse.

Of the twentieth-century psychological theories, the most discussed are those of Freud and his successors. Describing what he called the Oedipus complex, Freud wrote that a boy of four or five wants to have sex with his mother. The boy is afraid, according to Freud, that the father will discover this incestuous wish and castrate him. To defend himself, the boy either identifies with his father, becomes heterosexual, and thereby enjoys a vicarious sexual relationship with his mother, or he identifies with his mother and becomes homosexual.

Later psychoanalysts rejected Freud's theory, which was based on the belief that everyone is born bisexual and is potentially either heterosexual or homosexual. These sexist psychoanalysts were uncomfortable with the notion of bisexuality and proposed, instead, that boys are turned into homosexuals by "castrating" or "engulfing" mothers, women who are seductive toward their sons. Neither Freud's theory nor the later revisionist theory has the least bit of scientific evidence to support it, although this hasn't stopped the vast majority of psychoanalysts from trying to "cure" their homosexual patients.

By this point, it should be clear that there is no generally accepted theory to explain the origin of homosexuality. Researchers are still split between those who uphold either a psychological or a biological explanation. But is there any reason to "explain" the origins of homosexuality? Noticeably absent is any research into the etiology of heterosexuality. (Read *Homosexual Behavior: A Modern Reappraisal* by Judd Maimor and *Homosexuality: Research Implications for Public Policy* by John Gonsiorek and James Weinrich.)

Whenever society, through its medical authorities, has tried to "explain" homosexuality, such explanations have been merely pretexts for attempts to "cure" it. The cures have included castration, electric and chemical shock, imprisonment, and ostracism. Who can blame gays for being skeptical of the motives of straight authorities investigating the "etiology" of homosexuality? Don't let anyone try to change your sexual orientation. It's as natural as your need for food and drink. (Read *Cures* by Martin Duberman.)

NEW MACHO IMAGES

A glance at any old magazine or film shows that there has been a series of distinctive masculine looks. From decade to decade, there have always been men who managed to look both hot and handsome.

Why did men adopt these looks? Obviously, to be more attractive to others and, more specifically, as a sexual lure. Whether it's Johnny Motorcycle caressing his leather or Joe College hearing women sigh over the fit of his Dockers, men go out of their way to bait the hook to catch the fish of their choice. And when it's a gay man doing the baiting, he's got a head start: He knows what look, what fashion worn exactly how, turns *him* on. All he has to do is turn that around and do it to other guys.

The "clone" look of the seventies became the look most associated with gay men in the United States (indeed, around the world). It consisted of medium-length hair cut loose enough for a natural curl or wave, plus a beard and/or mustache. It was completed by a solidly muscled, well-tanned body that looked good in a Lacoste polo shirt with turned-up collar. Masculine was in, the more masculine the better.

The "butch gay" look was based on the black leather outfits of the S/M scene. Dark glasses and button-fly Levi's 501s, so tight they seemed painted on, were also a part of this image. These revealing denims were ideally worn with the Levi's top buttons open to show your perfect, rock-hard stomach. A pair of cowboy or engineer boots completed the ensemble.

Sound familiar? Cleaned up a bit, updated, splashed all over magazines and books, film and television, posed nude and seminude, this look became the standard macho style—from the Marlboro Man to Calvin Klein and Ralph Lauren ads to Chippendale's strip acts.

This stereotyped masculine image was in turn replaced by the "punk" look of the early eighties, which was too extreme for many and soon gave way to the post-club look, which means baggy clothing, clean-shaven face, and short hair. That didn't last long either, and all of these looks have now given way to a new amalgam, what we call the ACT UP clone, though many older gays are still comfortable with the previous style.

New macho images have also developed. among the most common of which are the Bear, the Wall Street Shark, and the gay yuppie (or guppie). The Bear has recently gotten much attention, with its own popular new magazine, meeting clubs, newsletters, and an entire line of clothing. The

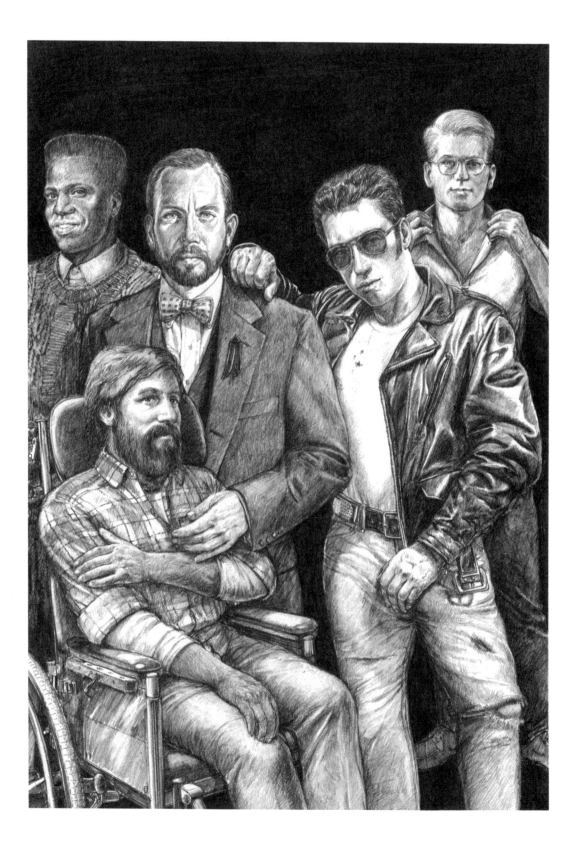

Bear look is all-natural, rural, even woodsy. Gone is the clipped neatness of the clone's facial hair: Full beards are common, as are bushy mustaches. Bears are stay-at-home wild men who enjoy football, trout fishing, carpentry, plumbing, and electrical repair work. They're just regular guys—only they're gay. The clothing, generally more countrified versions of the seventies clone's garb, says this, with its emphasis on wool workshirts, usually worn open over T-shirts or thermal knits, and wide belts with big buckles holding up torn-leg shorts or standard denims. Bears wear heavy hiking boots, with Pendleton shirt-jackets.

Bears are definitely hairy, often gray-haired. Their bodies are strong and masculine. They've got weight and are proud, even eager to show it. Big as their biceps and chests are, their stomachs are seldom washboards, their buttocks aren't disco cute. Everything about Bears is several hands fuller than usual. The Bear's urban variant is often seen in the leather bars.

The Wall Street Shark dresses and acts exactly as the name suggests— expensively, button-down English. He's pretty much indistinguishable from his hetero colleague—except, of course, he's gay. During the week, the Shark unwinds naturally into a more standard urban-suburban yuppie mode.

The guppie look reaches its apotheosis on the weekend, and the minute differences in this style vary geographically from resort to resort. Ralph Lauren has zeroed in on the shark/guppie look perfectly. His new lines of stone-washed twills, wide-wale corduroys, and denim pants, with equally worn-looking off-matching chambray, narrow-wale cord, and brushed-cotton shirts, accented by overlarge, knitted sweaters, unusually tinted mock turtlenecks, and mock sweat shirts, all covered by coats and jackets two sizes too large, all possess that ineffable look that guppies in the know love so well. It costs tons more than it looks.

For some reason it's not the guppie look so much as the Wall Street Shark look that has an irresistible attraction to its political opposite: the ACT UP clone.

Let's look at the ACT UP clone in detail. His hair is worn short, sometimes punkily long on top but cut so close at the sides it's nearly nonexistent. It is shaped into hints of eighties spikes, or clipped in little wedges that show up especially well when the hair is dyed a lighter color. For those without straight hair, bunches of curls are acceptable, as long as they're on the top of the head only. For others, a buzz cut reminiscent of the fifties crewcut is the ticket. Naturally, with so much emphasis placed on the head, facial hair is out, except for the little goatee, à la Lenin, or even just the triangle of hair under the lower lip. Sideburns are also verboten. Ditto body hair, which is generally clipped completely off, including the crotch area and especially any hair around the ass or on the balls (see *Shaving*).

The heavily muscled body seems to be becoming passé. Among whites the pasty look is in. Tanned is out. The aim is to look like a working-class high school student who's been left back a few times. Therefore, clothing is cheap, cheeky, and class conscious. Black Levi's are basic, worn tight at the ankle. Or, in warm weather, black denim or twill shorts are worn long and rolled up at the kneecaps. Shoes and boots are large, heavy, and clunky. Leather shoes tend to be hard-tipped lace-ups known as factory shoes, or, because of their cartoony shape, Sluggo shoes. These are worn with thick white socks. T-shirts tend to be regulation white. They are simple, cheap, pocketless, covered with political statements or portraits of little-known third-world personalities. More formal wear tends to long-sleeved, dark shirts, buttoned at the throat and wrists. Belts are multiple, with lots of metal—one of the few decorations in this outfit. Suspenders are commonly worn even with shorts and over T-shirts. Jackets can be simple leather, or off-the-rack black sport jackets, as shapeless as possible. Earrings are the invariable decoration. One earring is required: It can be a stud or ring. Two or more through an earlobe, one side of the nose, or a lip is not uncommon (see *Piercing*).

This look is a true rejection of the casual, leisure-class macho gay look. It does seem apt for all races—Asian, African-American, Latino, and Anglo (and thus it fits the ACT UP political agenda)—but less open to different physiques.

It remains to be seen whether this look will become more prevalent. Until that occurs, it will have to compete with other macho images—the clone, the Wall Street Shark, the guppie, and the Bear—in defining how gay men see and present themselves (see *Types*). As gays so totally influence fashion and design in our culture, our fashion of today will be worn by straight men next year.

NIBBLING AND BITING

Sensuality requires unpredictability. Once sex becomes routinized it loses its fascination, and just as a good conversationalist varies his tone, alternating humor with seriousness, small talk with big ideas, the full exposition with the abrupt transition, so in the same way a good lover keeps his partner slightly, wonderfully off balance. During a long, tender encounter, slow and dreamlike, a bite or a nibble can be the sudden flash of light amid the misty gray.

Your partner, say, is kissing you deeply, meditatively—but then he bites your lower lip in a short, sharp nip. Or he is licking every square inch of your body, from your forehead to your toes, but when he reaches the tender flesh on the inner side of your thighs just below your crotch he nibbles you playfully. Or you are alternately bathing his ear in saliva and blowing a cool stream of breath over the hot, wet skin—then you dive in to nibble his lobe.

Some people believe the ultimate is to nibble and worry one spot with a prolonged kiss, and leave a hickey there, something he must hide the next day with a high collar, but that he will see the following evening. Others

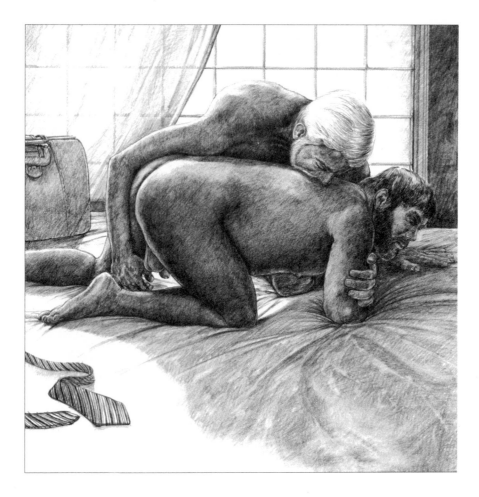

think hickeys too adolescent and prefer instead to nibble a partner's balls, nipples, and the cheeks of his ass. Each tastes different, and using lots of saliva while nibbling generally causes your partner to writhe in delight.

Obviously you need to be careful about any behavior that might puncture the skin and transmit HIV, but when that's not a problem, love bites add the proper spice to a sexual meal.

NIPPLES

One of the hottest sights around is a pair of ripe nipples on proud pecs bursting through a tight T-shirt. To get your pectorals just right you will have to go to the gym and sweat, but to achieve outstanding nipples, you can exercise right in your own home. Little by little, regular tit play will increase their size.

Doctors tell us that men and women have the same nerve endings in their nipples. In the last ten or fifteen years there has been more interest in tit play as gay men catch up on what women have always known: Your

ently, releases passion, in much the same way that flamenco dancers or gospel singers spur each other on to new heights of frenzy by shouting their excited approval.

If you're inhibited about vocalizing your pleasure, you might try this exercise with your partner: Let him masturbate you. You should not reciprocate for the moment, but rather concentrate on your own bodily sensations. Become conscious of your own breathing. Inhale deeply, and then when you exhale make a sound (as soft or as loud as you like). As your partner masturbates you, tell him what feels good. If you want him to go faster or slower along the shaft, tell him. As you become more and more excited, allow your vocalizations to become louder. The point is to express your feelings. And when you come, don't hold your breath. Make as much noise as you can on a single deep exhalation. You'll also notice, as you come out of your swoon, that your partner is in a fever of excitement and ready for his turn.

After you've had noisy sex a few times, you will probably make a few observations. First, vocalizing is a way of relaxing your diaphragm and throat and releasing your entire upper body. All too many people—used to furtive, silent sex—freeze the upper body and confine erotic sensations to below the belt. Second, you will learn that your vocalizations excite your partner and let him know, moment by moment, what you are feeling; this enhanced communication establishes greater intimacy.

Ethologists who study animal behavior in the wild have pinpointed many *innate releasing mechanisms*—reciprocal signals that mating animals send one another to trigger the next behavioral sequence in the sex act. No one knows for sure if the sounds of passion function this way in human beings, but at the very least, making noise seems to work in some analogous fashion. As your level of excitement rises, you make excited sounds, which in turn raise the level of your partner's passion until you are both caught in a reverberating cycle of pleasure.

ORGIES

Technically speaking, any time more than two people are having sex together an orgy is in progress. Over the years three-ways have become, if not common, then at least not unheard-of, especially in some long-term gay relationships (see *Three-ways*). However, there are usually more than three people at an orgy.

Most of our ideas about orgies derive from film. Biblical epics of the twenties, the thirties, and especially the Technicolorful fifties set the standard with their masses of writhing unclad and semiclad bodies, their "exotic" music, and their general sense of ambivalent anything-goes. Cecil B. DeMille was a filmmaker particularly skilled at displaying masses of seminude bodies within the context of a religious theme.

Like the best movies, the best orgies are carefully orchestrated in advance, and controlled throughout with occasional adjustments. Naturally, some orgies continue to be completely spontaneous, but these, alas, are few, far between, and all the more memorable for that rarity.

More than one gay youth has been astounded to discover that his presence (in a state of excitation if not undress) was all that was needed to begin an orgy among a group of men. Such "orgy flints" strike the appropriate sparks. But they're even rarer than spontaneity. As a result, organizing an orgy is difficult, at best. There are several ways to bring the participants together. If you're drop-dead handsome, or perfectly charming, or famous, or wealthy (or all four), and as a result, you have many (safe, we hope) sexual partners, simply invite them and tell them to bring along a horny friend. If your sexual tastes are very specific, you could end up with a room of six-foot blonds, all of whom like to fuck and refuse to get fucked. Paradise to you perhaps, but not to them. Or you can go out and round up likely candidates. You'll be surprised how flattered people are by the invitation, whether they accept or not. At Fire Island Pines, for example, the height of being in-with-the-in-crowd was the whispered invitation in your ear, one hour before the disco closed, to party at a local house known for its orgies: "Orgy at Surfside Six!"

Some gays get so many replies and phone calls to their sex ads they pool their respondents into a single date—i.e., an orgy (see *Sex Ads*). Others have become so adept at staging them that they throw an orgy once a week, which becomes a standing party to the initiated, and finally a local institution. These days, in larger cities, one finds semiprivate or pay-as-you-go clublike orgies staged every week (same time, same place) at someone's loft in the city or house in the hills.

Once everyone (or a quorum, at least) is assembled, the biggest problem is getting the orgy started. One way to break the ice is to greet your guests at the door naked, or in a jockstrap, or in underwear (torn, of course). Better yet, invite your most seductive friend to arrive early, and have him greet them. Another way is to instruct two or three lieutenants to start the ball rolling upon a prearranged cue.

Practical hints: Have plenty of liquid refreshments handy—although not necessarily liquor, which can lead to problems. If you're using your own home, it's a good idea to close off rooms you don't want invaded. Lock up your valuables, and place towels, lubricants, and condoms in conspicuous places. If you have strong feelings about the use of drugs, let people know about that in advance. Appropriate music can help an orgy succeed. Pop music shouldn't be too soft or sentimental. Quiet jazz (though not blues) and disco with its insistent, repetitive rhythms are good bets for sustaining a hot, pounding, sexual mood.

PARENTS

C oming out to parents can be difficult, especially if you are still living at home. The desire to come out to our parents is a measure of the growing self-esteem of gays. This wish is not only based upon a decision to be honest but also arises out of a need to communicate the good things that are happening in our lives.

A few tips about coming out at home: First, practice by coming out to some of your straight friends; study their reactions and examine how you feel as an out gay man. You should also ask your gay friends about their experiences coming out.

If you feel you want to come out to your parents, it's best to choose a moment when you are alone with them, away from brothers and sisters, and unlikely to be interrupted. Also, make sure that you choose a time when they are relaxed. During this discussion do not confuse the issue of homosexuality with other matters ("No wonder I'm gay, Dad, you never paid attention to me"). No blame attaches to anyone for your being gay, so you should not allow your parents to accuse themselves or each other. Nor should you allow them to blame you. Homosexuality is not something that needs to be blamed on anyone.

Your parents may accept your coming-out easily, or they may need a lot of time to accept your homosexuality. Be sure to give them all the information they require; you may be surprised how little they know. Your disclosure, however, is likely to stimulate worries they may have. Two of the most common questions are 1) Won't you be lonely? and 2) What are you doing to prevent getting AIDS? Be prepared to answer them. It's smart to get your folks a couple of books about homosexuality, especially those written specifically for parents. If there isn't a gay bookstore near you, get free catalogues from A Different Light Bookstore (800-343-4002) and Lambda Rising Bookstores (202-462-6969). Don't expect your parents to read the books immediately; they'll need time to work up the courage even to open them. You might also tell them about the nearest branch of Parents and Friends of Lesbians and Gays, a support group for parents. You can get a list of branches by writing to PFLAG, PO Box 27605, Washington, DC 20038. Since they're likely to feel shy about joining the group, you might offer to go with them. On the other hand, they might be uncomfortable if you accompany them, so don't feel resentful if they choose to go alone.

Your parents are going to need support and reassurance. Your news may come as a big surprise. Tell them you're disclosing your homosexuality to them because you love them and want to share this important area of your life. Tell them you're the same son you've always been. Tell them you love them; they need to hear you reaffirm your affection for them, since they have heard that homosexuals usually reject their families (a myth, but a common one). If they ask embarrassing details about your sex life (they usually don't want to know), just quietly tell them that yours is as private as theirs. You should accept the responsibility for telling your brothers and sisters you are gay; don't leave it to your parents.

Another dimension of coming out to parents is introducing your lover. More and more parents are accepting their sons' lovers, but one still finds some attacking the relationship, usually with the panicky rationalization that "he" made you gay, or if it weren't for "him" you'd marry that nice girl around the corner.

A visit to one's parents during a holiday is often the battleground for these skirmishes. "You're coming home *alone,* aren't you?" from a parent is not so much a question as it is a command, which usually means "Don't bring that bastard into *my* house!" Some gay men need their parents' approval so badly that they leave their lovers home. A different kind of gay man will say, "We're a couple, and we go places together. If that's not satisfactory, we won't visit you. Think it over and call me when you've decided what you want." Some gays find it helpful to invite recalcitrant parents to visit and meet a lover.

Often the difficulty comes from only one parent. Try to avoid playing one of them off the other, although naturally you'll want to enlist as much support as possible in helping you win acceptance from the recalcitrant parent. In some cases it's a sibling who reveals unsuspected depths of prejudice. This must be confronted. Don't worry that one or both parents will be so shocked that they will have a heart attack. That's an absurd notion. Your homosexuality cannot kill anyone. Even though it's anxiety-provoking, coming out to parents has its rewards. Not coming out to them cheats you out of that support.

In the past decade, AIDS or one's HIV status has increased the pressure on gay men to divulge their homosexuality to their parents. A seropositive gay man may no longer want to hide his life-style, because he hears a clock ticking. There are also gay men who have come out to their parents only after being diagnosed with HIV Disease. The most conflict-laden scene occurs when a gay man lying mortally ill in a hospital tells his parents he is gay and simultaneously that he has contracted AIDS. This is a classic double whammy. As a son, recognize how difficult this will be for your parents to absorb, and help them by directing them to friends, social workers, or medical staff who can answer many of the questions they're sure to have (see *Body Positive; HIV Disease*).

The HIV crisis has confirmed what we know about parents and their capacity for love. The majority of parents respond with compassion for their sons. They support their sons emotionally, financially, and physically. So do siblings. These parents have also recognized the value of their sons' lovers and friends, who share the burden of caring for the ill son, cooking, washing, and crying with him. In these cases, parents, lovers, and friends also provide important support for each other.

Unfortunately, not all parents are loving people. In fact, a shocking number of them have turned out to be selfish and narcissistic in their reactions to the AIDS crisis. "How could he have done this *to me?*" is a typical comment from such a parent. They totally abandon their sons. They refuse to visit sons who are dying; they refuse to phone or to write. Frantic calls from the son's lover or from other family members are ignored. If a sick son wants to visit them they refuse to see him.

After the son's death, these selfish parents swoop down and steal his body without informing the son's lover or friends, the very people who cared for him throughout his illness. They dispose of it in a private ceremony, so that they won't be embarrassed by a funeral. They certainly don't attend the memorial services held by the lover or the friends of the deceased. Often, their final revenge on their son for his homosexuality is to violate the terms of his will.

The HIV crisis has not created these monsters; they were there all the time. But AIDS has forced us to rethink our relationship to our parents. We are reminded that some parents do not love their children and possibly never loved them—or anyone else, for that matter.

Some gay sons should *not* come out to their parents—ever; they should refuse to have anything to do with them. This is not said lightly. Gay men who come from spiteful families must (and doubtless will) seek support and love elsewhere, because in their cases, love never has and never will come from their parents. It's hard enough to give up parents when they die; oddly, it appears to be even more painful emotionally to give up unloving parents. Perhaps it's terrifying to realize that you were right about them all the time.

PHONE SEX

Ma Bell has gone into the sex business. Every gay newspaper and magazine has advertisements featuring hunky models with big dicks encouraging you to phone them. For just a dollar or two a minute (just?!), you'll find a dreamboat of a man who's impatiently waiting for you. Thousands of men call every day for two reasons: Some want only to jerk off, others to meet men.

Jerking off on the phone has many advantages over real life. Obviously one doesn't have to look one's best, and there's no need to worry about unsafe sex. Probably the most reassuring aspect is the safety of anonymity. Phone sex is not threatening, and while one can be rejected by other callers, the rejection seems not to hurt so much as it does face-to-face. There's always someone else to talk to. With the fear of rejection diminished, gay men are free to use their imaginations, in fact free to stretch them to the limit.

Phone sex might even teach you about some aspects of the mysteries of Eros that you have never thought about before. Do you love light, boyish voices and turn off to deep, masculine tones that smack of your father's cold authoritarianism—or do you tremble and grow weak in the knees when a guy's deep voice has the comforting authority of Walter Cronkite's? Do Midwestern accents fill you with thoughts of rolling around in a rustling field with a cornsilk-blond farm boy, even though the body attached to the voice may be that of a WASP who works in a three-piece suit? Do sleepy slow Southern voices summon up visions of long lazy nights of tender lovemaking, or do they turn you off, irrationally but inevitably, making you think about homophobic rednecks?

There's no truth in advertising on the phones. Almost everyone entices with exaggerated descriptions of themselves. Any cock that measures from four to seven inches will be described as eight inches long; it'll be cut or uncut, depending upon what the owner thinks you want to hear. If it's actually eight inches, the proud possessor will boldly proclaim it a nine- or ten-inch whammer. He may even have given his cock a name in honor of its imposing size, although no one to our knowledge has yet cataloged the nicknames of people's peckers. Just as additions are made to cock size, subtractions are made from age. The general rule appears to be a five-year discount, so a thirty-year-old claims to be twenty-five, and so on up the line. On the other hand, young guys, from the teens to the young twenties, sometimes increase their age by a few years in order not to frighten away older gentlemen (in their thirties).

Other physical descriptions are equally inaccurate. A man who describes himself as a football player is probably overweight. The caller's claim to have a swimmer's body may be interpreted to mean that he's thin, perhaps very thin—quite unlike swimmers' bodies these days.

All this exaggeration, and blatant lying, is perfectly all right, even preferable, if your intention is to jerk off on the phone. Under these circumstances, don't let your usual inhibitions stand in the way of describing yourself as the perfect man, whatever that may mean to you. Both you and your caller will be the better for it. And of course don't even allow yourself to wonder whether the description he's given you is accurate. It's all fantasy, make-believe, just for fun, just to get a load off.

On the other hand, you may be the kind of person who wants to meet people through the phone lines. In this case, we advise you to describe yourself accurately to your phone mate. If you're standing in the rain at three A.M. ringing someone's doorbell, and you've described yourself over the phone as looking like Tom Cruise, although you more accurately resemble Henry Kissinger, don't expect to get in. It makes no sense to lie about yourself if you want to meet men over the phone. In the first place, such lying indicates that you're insecure about some physical characteristic. This turns people off. In the second place, you may find someone on the phone who is aroused by the very thing that turns you off about yourself. Find him, and you'll not only have a good time, but you'll end up feeling better about yourself.

It makes a difference at what time you call. Let's take weekdays first. Seven A.M. to 9:00 A.M. is jerk-off time. That's when you'll likely hear someone say, "Can I take care of your morning load?" Then it's off to work like everyone else. The afternoon can also be jerk-off time, but with a different group of people. That's when the horny artists, free-lancers, and waiters, frustrated with their work, take to the phones. Early evening is slump time for phone sex. People are going about their business, meeting friends, having dinner, or going to the movies. Prime time is 11:00 P.M. to 2:00 A.M. These are "the relentless hours." Men call at this time because they want something hot before bed. Many men do not enjoy standing around in smoky bars drinking beer after beer, so they use the phone to meet each other. In other words, prime time is more about meeting than about jerking off.

From 2:00 A.M. to 6:00 A.M. you may get people who have been partying all night on drugs and alcohol. They call because their desires are artificially heightened. Because of the drugs, they can't get hard-ons and they make for rather dreary sex in person, but not necessarily over the phone. The post-club crowd, high on Ecstasy, are also on the line at this time. So much for weekdays.

Weekend nights on the phone are often not about phone sex, but about making contact and setting up a meeting. Phone lines are at a premium on weekend nights, and busy signals are common. The phone lines are also used by couples looking for a third party to spice things up at home.

If you invite someone over to your apartment and you've never met before, look through your peephole to make certain only one person shows up. If there's more than one, don't let them in, unless you planned it that way. Some men believe that they reduce risks by going over to the other man's house. Others prefer a neutral place such as a streetcorner or coffee shop so they can see and talk with the guy before bringing him home.

The actual procedure for using a phone line is simple enough. Dial the number. You'll probably get a recorded message asking whether you prefer a one-to-one or group line. The message should also tell you the cost. (If it doesn't, hang up immediately. Caveat emptor!) You'll then hear a beep, which means you've been connected. Start talking, perhaps saying "What's up?" or "What are you looking for?" Someone will respond. You want to find out a number of things. You want to know whether he's interested in jerking off or meeting. If you both want to meet, find out where he lives, since you may or may not want to go to his neighborhood, or it may take too much time to travel there. You want to know what he's into, the type of sexual scene that turns him on and whether it's compatible with your own. You may also want to know what he's wearing. Attire, or lack of it, is extremely important for those into jocks, underwear, or leather.

To reduce phone bills (which can reach astronomical heights if you're not careful) some men give out their phone numbers. If you do, be prepared to get calls *at any time of the day or night.*

Attitude is important. Nastiness or aggressiveness over the phone is ordinarily rewarded with hang-ups. On the other hand, sounding like a top or being authoritative may be just the thing your phone mate is looking for. Be very verbal. Use a lot of adjectives describing yourself and your favorite sexual scenes. Your descriptions should help the other man conjure up an image. Goose it all up with a sexy-sounding voice. If your voice is high, practice talking with a hushed, low voice.

As one man said, "The come-audio is very important." Since you can't actually see each other ejaculate, the sounds you make will vivify the images for your phone partner. Turn the sound up! If you come gently in real life, make it sound like an explosion over the phone. If your come just dribbles out in real life, make believe it hits the walls or squirts all over your face. And coming over the phone should take much longer than it does in actuality. These exaggerations make it all the more fun.

Along the way some people may hang up on you. Don't be offended or take it personally. The nicest people will say good-bye, but others won't take the time, and on the phones, time is money. The hang-up is probably only because you don't fit the other person's fantasy, or because he wants to meet someone who lives in his own neighborhood.

Is using phone lines harmful, psychologically speaking? If you use them to get your rocks off from time to time, then it's just a minor diversion and not a problem. But phone sex can become a persistent and expensive habit, especially if it's preventing you from meeting other gay men and forming love relationships. Jerking off on the phone can also become so specialized that it interferes with establishing a face-to-face relationship. If you cannot integrate phone fantasies into romantic relationships, or if persistent use of phone lines prevents the establishment of emotional attachment, you should probably avoid them. After all, while you can hang up on a person on the phones, you can't settle a conflict with a person right in front of you—date or lover—that way. Settling a conflict with someone you care about means exposing your emotional vulnerability, one type of behavior fastidiously avoided on the phones.

Don't fall into the trap of using the phone as a way to avoid intimacy or to evade real human companionship. The trials and tribulations involved in actually meeting guys face-to-face and crotch-to-crotch can be avoided by using the phone lines, but don't forget the phone is just an inanimate object and in the long run no substitute for cuddling, kissing, sucking, fucking, and a real live beating human heart.

PIERCING

Piercing body parts has a long history. For example, Caesar's body-guards were said to have worn nipple rings as a sign of their virility. In ancient America, ritual piercing was practiced by the Maya and other cultures. Sculptures show cords studded with thorns being passed

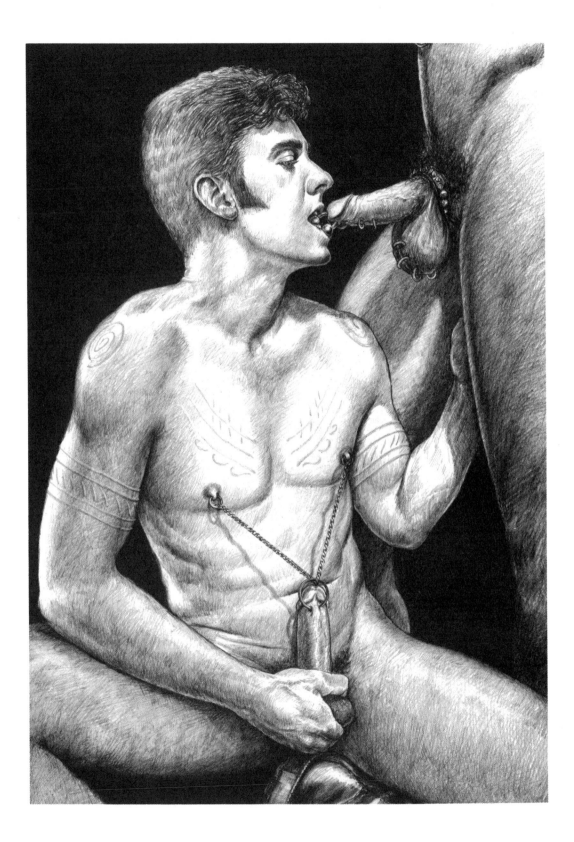

through the tongue or penis. This was a religious rite related both to fertility and penitence.

Seventeenth-century buccaneers often pierced their ears and wore a gold piece, sometimes a coin taken from the treasure hold of some hapless galleon that had fallen captive. Each earring commemorated a ship the pirate had helped capture. German U-boat sailors during World War I also marked their "kills" in this fashion.

What goes on here? Piercing is but one form of body decoration, a practice that also includes tattooing and scarification. Devotees of piercing explain that it is like tattooing, whose practitioners treat the human body as a canvas upon which colorful art is etched. In piercing, the human body serves as an armature to which metal sculpture is attached.

More recently, during the eighties, earrings joined tattoos and wildly carved and dyed hair as signs that set one apart. Of all the punk body-fashions, piercing and rings are the only ones to have been assimilated by the larger society. In gay urban centers, many men wear a single ring or stud in one ear. Two, three, or more rings are not uncommon, either thin gold rings an eighth of an inch apart near the center of the lobe, or a series of rings around the entire curved edge of the ear. In these examples piercing is a fashion statement. Earrings, nose rings, lip rings, eyebrow rings, and in some cases even tit rings have no sexual meaning.

Sexual piercing, on the other hand, is generally a component of S/M sex (see *Sadomasochism*). It, too, seems to have become more popular over the past decade. Was it always there—in the closet, so to speak? Probably.

Most S/M piercing is done on and around the cock. In the very popular *Prince Albert,* the head of the cock is pierced through the urethra, and a ring is inserted. The *guiche* (pronounced "geesh") is a piercing through the perineum, the space between the balls and the asshole. A neat chastity device can be made by locking a Prince Albert to a guiche. The *frenum* is a piercing through the frenum of the cock (the loose piece of flesh beneath the cock head). Tit piercing is also extremely common. There are other variations of cock piercing and ball piercing, and a sophisticated terminology is associated with them.

A variety of jewelrylike devices can be placed through these pierced holes. Rings and barbell studs are probably the most common. D rings, clamps, and locks are other forms of adornment. Most of this jewelry is made of surgical steel, although some men prefer gold. Some gay couples symbolize their relationship by means of a ritual piercing. They wear their rings on their cocks instead of on their fingers.

The act of piercing or the use of rings or studs may be the whole of the sexual experience between the partners. Sucking and fucking, so common in most other forms of sex, may or may not be part of the piercing scene. Some men will jerk off, while others may not come at all.

Piercing may also be temporary, in contrast to the placement of rings and studs. For instance, one expert places needles in the body of his partner, then connects them with kite string to form a frame above the body. Combining piercing with bondage, he then "plays the instrument," plucking the strings to create pain in different parts of the body. The object of this, according to S/M experts, is to reach what they call the *pleasure/pain threshold*. This is the point at which the body changes the perception of pain to a perception of pleasure. S/M practitioners believe that this is a biochemical process caused by the production of endorphins as a reaction to the pain. There is not yet scientific evidence to confirm or refute this claim.

There are obvious dangers to be avoided. Never pierce yourself, and never allow a stranger to pierce you. Piercing should only be done by professionals who have the proper sterile equipment and who can advise you about aftercare, which can last from two to six months. You might consult the Gauntlet, Inc., with stores in San Francisco, Los Angeles, and New York.

Drummer magazine for men and *On Our Backs* for lesbians carry ads from professional piercers.

PLEASURE TRAP

A man caught in the pleasure trap is willing to give pleasure to others but does not seek his own sexual satisfaction. He says he doesn't mind if he doesn't have an orgasm; all he wants to do is make you feel good. In tricking, such a person seems an ideal partner, completely unselfish and giving. But in a long-term relationship his refusal to express his own needs becomes (or at least is perceived as) a form of hostility. A relationship always implies reciprocity, and the man caught in the pleasure trap refuses to allow reciprocity.

What causes some men to give but not take gratification? They may be attempting to blackmail their partners into loving them by acting so unselfishly; the unconscious bargain they are proposing is "I will satisfy your sexual needs if you will take care of my emotional ones." Or they may be afraid to feel the full force of their sexual impulses, fearing that if these needs were ever unleashed they would become all-devouring. Or they may suffer from poor self-esteem or body image, believing that they don't deserve sexual pleasure and surely don't have the right to ask for it (see *Body Image; Guilt*). Or they may be martyrs, hoping to demonstrate their long-suffering patience (and thereby manipulate their partners). There are also men who suffer from the pleasure trap because of their own homophobic self-hatred.

Whatever the origin of this problem, it *is* a problem and should be treated. Not only does it cheat both partners out of the thrill of mutual sex, but it also causes the afflicted individual to feel alienated from his own body. Working with a lover on the problem can help, though most people will need to enter psychotherapy.

PORNOGRAPHY

But I warn you, with yet more solemn emphasis, against EVIL BOOKS and EVIL PICTURES. There is in every town an undercurrent which glides beneath our feet, unsuspected by the pure; out of which, notwithstanding, our sons scoop many a goblet. Books are hidden in trunks, concealed in dark holes; pictures are stored in sly portfolios, or trafficked from hand to hand; and the handiwork of depraved art is seen in other forms which ought to make a harlot blush. . . .

So wrote Henry Ward Beecher about the dangers of pornography. Even earlier, in 1675, a group of young dons at All Souls College were caught using the Oxford University presses to print copies of Giulio Roman's engravings of Aretino's *Postures,* the most famous, possibly the only, illustrated sex manual of the day. We don't know what punishment they were given for their pornographic (or commercial) interest. And in 1889, the novelist Henry James writes in a letter of some sadness that young men in front of him at Westminster Abbey were passing around photographs of naked Italian men at a memorial service for the poet Robert Browning.

Gay porn is divided into soft-core and hard-core. Soft-core consists of photos of men dressed, partly dressed, or naked, but usually alone and without erections. Hard-core pornography, on the other hand, consists of photographs, stories, films, or videotapes of guys masturbating, fucking, sucking, and actively engaging in sex. Besides rental videos, porn can be found at porno theaters, on TVs at some bars, sex clubs, baths, and private parties.

The object of pornography is to turn you on. Most people use pornography to excite themselves to a point where they will either jerk off or have sex with a partner. In fact, lovers often use pornography as a prelude to having sex together. Some feminists claim that pornography has another purpose, i.e., to demean women, while right-wingers say that porno is designed to destroy the nuclear family. These groups have their own political agendas. It is, however, true that men are more easily aroused sexually by visual means than most females are; whether this is biological or the result of socialization is still debated.

Almost anything can become pornography. An underwear or swimsuit ad in a magazine, an International Male catalog, even an ad for beer or a soft drink can be arousing. Some are turned on by drawings in which specific physical details (rounded buns, big cocks, massive chests) have been emphasized. Many young boys get their first glimpse of nudity by thumbing through old *National Geographic*s, conveniently found in most school libraries.

Videos, however, are the area where gay pornography has become most sophisticated. Gone are the days of amateurishly shot, grainy black-and-white 16mm flicks. In the late seventies, *Boys in the Sand* and *Bijou* were

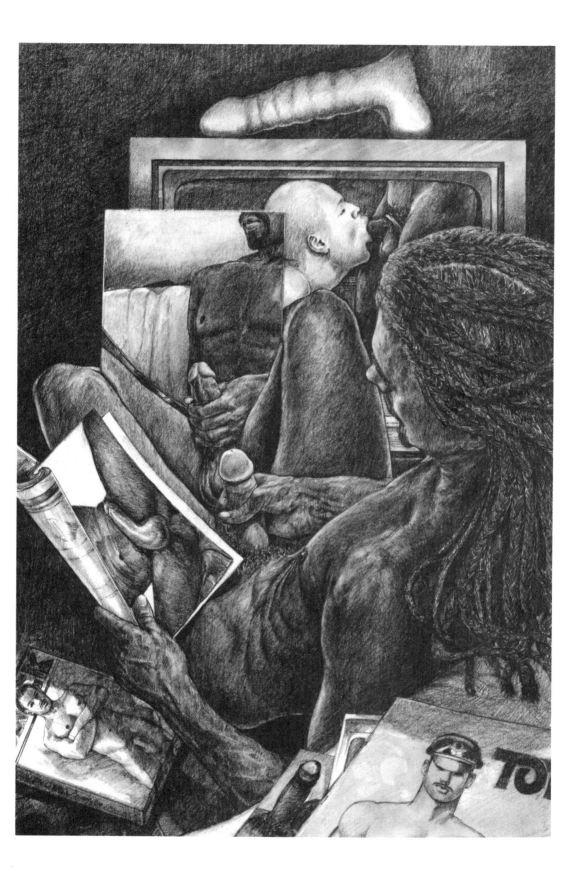

among the best-made porno films. Later, filmmakers like Kristin Bjorg went to Brazil to make porn and brought back an entire new range of physical types. Other filmmakers, like Christopher Rage, concentrated on kinkier stuff; his films remain the cutting edge. Joe Gage and Fred Halstead concentrated on making beautiful films using gorgeous guys in all kinds of scenes. Videotapes have now all but replaced films, and a whole new collection of porn stars has been acclaimed.

Few videos or photographs leave much to the imagination, and as a result, some men turn to written pornography. The very fact that the protagonists' looks are only suggested can be a real stimulant to the imagination. A whole line of unillustrated quickie gay novels is available in most pornography shops, and there is an entire series of true-stories anthologies of gay sexual experiences from military scenes to boarding schools, prisons, and travel. The best of these books (edited by Boyd McDonald) are sold under titles like *Filth, Smut,* and *Meat,* and contain relevant photos, mostly of either young blue-collar semi-hustlers or bodybuilders from the American Model Guild. At their best, these books are not only sexy, they're informative, intriguing, politically and socially savvy.

The only psychological disadvantage to pornography is that it could easily give rise to unreasonable expectations and dissatisfaction with the looks and performance of a sex partner. Can real life live up to Technicolor? In the constant interplay between the need for intimacy and the need for fantasy, neither should crowd out the other.

PROBLEMS OF EJACULATION

There are two kinds of ejaculatory problems—*premature ejaculation* (coming too fast) and *retarded ejaculation* (inability to come at all). While people with retarded ejaculation exercise too much control over their sexual responses, those afflicted by premature ejaculation lack control—or rather, have too little awareness of their bodily cues. A man who ejaculates prematurely is not aware of what's happening in his cock and the muscles surrounding it.

One self-help technique for coming too fast is this: Choose an understanding partner to jerk you off to the point of coming. Concentrate on your sensations and be on the alert for signals of imminent ejaculation. When you think you're about to come, tell your partner to stop masturbating you. Once the urge to come has abated, ask him to start jerking you off again. Once more stop him when you're close to climax. Repeat this exercise twice more; then go ahead and come.

During the next class (school was never like this!) your partner sucks you off to a point just short of climax. When you feel you're about to come, stop him. Repeat three times, then come. The final step is fucking.

When fucking, the best way to start out is with your partner on top (see *Sitting on It*). He should make slow movements up and down on your cock while you concentrate on your own physical sensations. When you feel that orgasm is near, stop him. Repeat three times. On the fourth time, go ahead and come. After you have overcome premature ejaculation in this position, you can switch to the side-by-side position (see *Side by Side*). Remember, always go slowly. Safe sex guidelines should be followed during these exercises.

Men who suffer from retarded ejaculation perform adequately until it's time to come—and then they can't. They usually have no problem coming while jerking off in the privacy of their bedrooms. For other men there's no problem in coming when someone else jerks them off or sucks them off, but they have trouble when fucking.

The immediate physical cause of retarded ejaculation, it's thought, is involuntary muscular overcontrol. The muscles around the genitalia appear to lock shut and there is nothing you can do about it, since they are under the control of the autonomic (involuntary) nervous system. It's a common response in men who are extremely tired (as is impotence). It may also occur in a man who's been fucking for a long time, but trying not to come. He may succeed all too well. In these cases the problem is situational, not chronic.

The deeper, psychological cause, however, is probably anxiety. Fear of sex, guilt about homosexuality, anxiety about pleasing one's partner—all these are possible factors. A number of psychologists suggest there may also be a strong unconscious hostile element involved. Whether anxiety is channeled into impotence, or retarded ejaculation, or the inability to get fucked depends upon one's psychological makeup. An impotent man will become flooded with anxiety; a late comer, by contrast, probably doesn't feel anxious.

If retarded ejaculation is persistent and long-standing, this exercise should help. If you have no problem masturbating alone, be sure to continue your jerk-off sessions. One evening ask someone you can completely trust to sit in the next room while you jerk off to orgasm. The next night invite him to sit in the next room while you masturbate for a few minutes. As you approach climax, he should enter the room, but not look at you. The next day he should come in the room while you're jerking off, at first with his back to you, the next time facing you.

Stagy and contrived as this procedure might sound, it follows a sound principle—psychologists call it *desensitization*. In any set of desensitization exercises you start with a situation that provokes no anxiety, then slowly move, step by step, toward the situation that alarms you. In overcoming retarded ejaculation, you are moving from jerking off alone, a relaxed situation, to jerking off in front of a partner. Once jerking off with him in the room and facing you is comfortable, he should come closer, and just as you are about to climax, he should take over and masturbate you.

Late comers habitually study themselves and watch their partners for reactions. This scrutiny only makes the problem worse. Turn out the light and surrender yourself to your fantasies. Forget about your cock, forget about what your partner is thinking, and picture a mouth-watering scene. If no fantasy springs to mind, use pornography. As you get caught up in this distracting whirl, your partner should jerk you off to climax. On the next evening he should go through the same procedure. Finally, try fucking him after you're midway through jerking yourself off.

Psychotherapy is not especially recommended for ejaculation problems, although sex therapy may be useful. Find out the name of a professional sex therapist and consult him or her. If you and your lover have become anxious in your attempts to cope with the problem, you may both welcome the assistance of an objective third person.

PROMISCUITY

The word "promiscuity" is usually used pejoratively, in such loaded statements as "The AIDS crisis is a direct result of promiscuity in the gay community." It's not a neutral description but a moral condemnation, and is used against gays by any group that condemns homosexuality. What constitutes promiscuity depends upon the speaker and his value system. One person will call a man who has two sexual partners promiscuous; another will reserve this condemnation for a regular frequenter of brothels. As a rule, gay men call someone promiscuous if he has a lot of sex with a lot of different guys.

Such a man is often called a slut or a whore because he has a bigger appetite than the rest of us. People say he is promiscuous because he won't "grow up" and "settle down" with a lover. Interestingly enough, the word "promiscuous" is seldom applied to those gay men who have a chain of relationships over a period of years—what's usually called serial monogamy.

The word "promiscuous" should be retired from the vernacular. As a rule of thumb, if a gay man is unattached there's no harm in his having as much (safe) sexual experience as he wants. If he has a lover, they should decide how much sex, if any, they want outside their relationship, and under what circumstances (see *Couples; Fidelity and Monogamy; Jealousy, Envy, and Possessiveness*). One lover having sex without the other's knowledge is not promiscuous but dishonest; this situation is best viewed as a failure of communication rather than a moral flaw.

On the other hand, there are men whose obsession with sex is so severe that it threatens to take over their lives. Sexual desire becomes the tail that wags the dog, and these men's lives are disrupted by the incessant search for sex, regardless of place or time, regardless of the partner or the pleasure. This runaway sex can interfere significantly with their work and social life.

pieces. Often the same African-American or Latino who is received cordially when accompanied by a white person is carded when he's alone. In establishments where carding takes place, black or Asian-American couples at "Anglo" places are virtually always carded. In this way, people are, at the very least, hassled. Even if permitted to enter, they have been made to feel unwanted and unwelcome. At the worst, they're discriminated against and kept out.

We call the exclusion of *any* race or ethnic group by *any* other race or ethnic group racism. We believe African-Americans who exclude Asian-Americans, and Latinos who exclude African-Americans are as racist as whites who exclude blacks, though the latter is by far the most common form of racism in our society.

Some gay men worry that their sexual interest (or lack of it) in blacks and Latinos may be racist. We think not (see *Types*). On the other hand, white men who sleep with blacks and Latinos but who then exclude them socially *are* expressing racist attitudes.

RAPE

In recent years, the incidence of rape of men by men has increased significantly. In fact, many cases of rape are forms of gay-bashing, perpetrated by straight men (often in groups) against gay men.

Feminists and sociologists have called our society a culture of rape. Its characteristics are sexual inequality, exploitation of sex in commerce and entertainment, and rigid concepts of sin and retribution. The attacker invariably blames the victim by saying that she or he dressed, acted, or spoke "provocatively," or in some other way "asked for it."

"Rape is about power, not about sex" has become a commonly heard statement. Yet sex and power are intimately related. What changes sexual intercourse (in its widest sense) into rape is not the force used, but rather the lack of consent.

Which leads to one of the dirty secrets of recent gay life: *date rape*. This used to be rare among men, often the result of crossed signals. An experienced man, for instance, might pick up someone who was just coming out and, misled by the inexperienced one's flirtatiousness, think he wants to have sex. In fact, however, the inexperienced one is just looking for conversation and cuddling. The experienced man may fail to respect his partner's limits. Overcome by a combination of resentment and lust, he may force sex on his partner.

The increased frequency of date rape in recent years seems to be directly related to the fear many gays feel about contracting HIV Disease. Less willing to be sexually active, yet attracted to their partner, they appear indecisive; another may interpret the indecision as flirting. Should the misunderstanding continue, the partner may feel frustrated. If he has a violent streak in his personality, sexual assault may be the result.

Rape has always occurred in prisons. Many male prisoners force weaker or younger men to serve as substitutes for women. In recent years, potential victims have been placed in special cell blocks to decrease the incidence of rape. Unless segregated, the younger, slighter, more attractive male in prison better be ready to defend his asshole.

Rape is assault and can produce physical as well as psychological harm. If you have been raped, you should report it to the police and seek medical care, even though cops may be unsympathetic to a gay man. Many larger cities have rape crisis lines you can call. They can advise you about how to handle the police and get medical treatment, and where to seek counseling. If such crisis lines or clinics do not exist in your area, check your local gay center or gay info hot line. Ask to talk to someone who can refer you for treatment. You can always call the New York City Gay and Lesbian Anti-Violence Project twenty-four hours a day at 212-807-0197.

Seek medical treatment whether you report the rape or not. This may include a rectal exam to check for internal tears or bleeding. Usually it's done by hospital staff connected with a rape center. You might also want to be monitored over the following weeks for disease (see *Sexually Transmitted Diseases*).

An even more painful kind of gay rape occurs when a father (or step-father) sexually assaults his son. There may be anal or oral penetration. These assaults often begin before puberty, and may continue for years. Sons who have been sexually assaulted by a parent (occasionally it's a mother) are terrified of divulging the secret. They are often rightly afraid of paternal violence against themselves or other members of the family. Particularly reprehensible parents will threaten to kill the child's pet if they tell.

If you have been raped by your father, don't keep it a secret any longer. You owe it to yourself to confront the problem. You also owe it to siblings who may still be at home. Find someone you can talk to, perhaps a teacher or a friend's parents; definitely see a psychotherapist. If a friend confides information like this to you, be compassionate and guide him to people or organizations that can help. You might want to read *Victims No Longer* by Mike Lew (Harper & Row, 1988, 1990).

Gay men also have fantasies about being raped, but these are quite different from the foregoing acts of exploitation. Gay men sometimes masturbate to the fantasy that another man (or the entire college football team) is forcing sex upon him. Some find the scenario arousing, and even act it out with tricks or lovers. There's also a large collection of pornography based upon these ideas. Don't feel guilty if you enjoy the fantasy. It doesn't mean that you want to be really raped. Part of the fun in gay life seems to be the ability to let go during sexual fantasies, and to become passive in the arms of another man. The "rape," we suspect, is but a transformation of the desire to be taken care of by another man.

REJECTION

Being rejected by a particular stranger in a particular bar on a Tuesday night at eleven-thirty P.M. is not a final judgment on whether or not you are attractive. Look at the event objectively. Ask yourself what his reasons might have been. He might be tired, have a cold, or have a lover waiting for him at home. Perhaps he's just finished having sex, or you're not his type because you have a beard (or because you don't). There's no way you can ascertain his motives, but bear in mind that they may have nothing to do with you (see *Types*). Try to remember all those who said yes to you over the years, as well as your achievements, both personal and professional.

How should you handle hurt feelings when someone turns you down? Since no one gets used to rejection, there's likely to be a momentary shock.

There are three responses that should be avoided:

1. Immediately finding fault with the man who rejected you: "He's not so great" or "I'm sure that tan is out of a bottle." Revenge or spite only serves to keep you obsessed with a rejection best forgotten.

2. Going around rejecting others. Having been shot down, you decide to put a few notches on your own gun. After letting someone squirm until he works up the courage to ask you home, you have the (perfectly hollow) pleasure of rejecting him.

But the worst response is:

3. Depression. You indulge in self-pity. You decide that your personality is dull, your looks are repellent, and your life is meaningless. You have five more drinks and then stagger home, feeling old, ugly, and hopeless.

If rejection is so wounding, you should ask yourself what past experiences you may be unconsciously reliving—rejection by a parent, a childhood friend, or first lover. One occasionally finds men who are very accomplished at setting themselves up for rejection by picking out the coldest man in the bar, the one most likely to turn them down. Such a self-defeating pattern of behavior needs to be faced squarely and dealt with in therapy or self-analysis.

Perhaps it's time for a change, time to move on to a new spot, a new meeting place, and a new group of people. You'll be surprised how being a new face can pick up your social life and cut down rejection. On the other hand, maybe you do need to make some changes in yourself. Make an honest evaluation of your behavior in social situations. Perhaps your anxiety is being expressed in a hostile or rigid attitude. If so, change this. We have all to make adjustments in ourselves from time to time.

RELAXATION

S ometimes people become overwhelmed with anxiety just before or during sex. If you have this problem, take time to relax. Although you may fear your partner will be insulted if you don't jump right into sex with him, he may welcome the opportunity to enjoy a breather himself. In most cases, vulnerability is more appealing than you'd suspect.

One relaxation technique is, paradoxically, to tighten sets of muscles deliberately. Start with your hands. Make them into fists, then open them and say to yourself, "Relax." Next, tighten your arms and then relax them. Pay special attention to the tension in your neck and stomach. Throughout your exercises breathe deeply. Psychologists call this *progressive relaxation*.

Another technique is to call to mind a scene that is totally calm, maybe one out of your past or, alternatively, one you have made up. It might be a beach or a forest or a picture-book castle, but whatever it is, if you tune in to it, it will create a relaxed physical condition.

You might ask your partner to help you. Lie very still, trying to relax your body as much as possible. Imagine i. is so heavy it will sink through the bed, or so limp that you are like a rag doll. Then your partner should pick up your hand or foot and drop it back to the bed. Alternatively, you can lie back, concentrate on breathing deeply, and have your partner massage you as you exhale. Each time you breathe in you should be able to inhale more easily and more deeply.

Once you are fully relaxed, you can ease into sex. If, however, during the course of sexual activity you become anxious again, don't be afraid to stop for another breather. *Taking the time to relax is much sexier than being tense during lovemaking.*

RIMMING

T hough often used as a preliminary to fucking, rimming is fun in itself and an effective way to relax the muscles of the asshole. Unfortunately, rimming is also an easy way to contract several serious diseases, including hepatitis A, amebiasis (and other parasitic diseases), and venereal diseases, such as syphilis and gonorrhea (see *Sexually Transmitted Diseases*).

There is no evidence to prove that rimming, or being rimmed, has transmitted HIV, but doctors are unsure about it as a route of transmission. Therefore, rimming is clearly considered an unsafe sex practice. It should not be practiced with tricks since their sexual history is unknown to you. Do it only when you are absolutely certain of the health status of your sexual partner.

Using dental dams, thin plastic squares used to protect the mouth during orthodontic surgery, is sometimes recommended. Don't use Saran Wrap or the like. It's porous and won't prevent disease.

Here's how to rim. Gently run your fingers along the curves of your partner's back until you reach the buns. Knead and cup them; just barely touch the crack. Knead your partner's cheeks and give him a few light nips with your teeth. Some men like to slap their partners' buns at this point so as to heighten his excitement. Run your fingers down the crack, and draw a line with your tongue all the way to his balls.

Reach between his legs and play with his cock. Simultaneously work your tongue into the crack of his ass. Lick a circle, making smaller and smaller arcs until the tongue can feel the difference between the skin around the hole and the muscle. Dart and flicker in and out.

Rimming can be done in many different positions. Your partner can be on his back with his legs in the air. You can be in a sixty-nine position (see *Sixty-nining*), you sucking your partner's cock while he rims you. Or he can be flat on his stomach, while you feast between his buttocks (see *Sit on My Face*).

Rimming can be passionate; the man rimming feels his partner's ass contract and relax, which spurs him on. The man being rimmed can push back toward the tongue or rotate his hips. He'll sigh; his breathing will come faster and sharper—responses that usually delight his partner, and encourage him to new efforts.

ROLE-PLAYING

In the past, there were psychological advantages to social role-playing. It reduced anxiety by defining social behaviors: "You do the dishes, I take out the garbage. You invite the guests, I support the family." Role-playing, therefore, established ground rules governing the relationship between two people.

Today, such role-playing scarcely works even for heterosexuals, although they have been carefully coached from childhood on what constitutes proper male and female behavior. The gay couple has no stake in preserving the male-female social dichotomy.

Sexual role-playing is something different. A gay man may decide to assume a specific but temporary sexual role. On one occasion, he may want to dominate a cute "kid," and the next night he may want to be the kid himself. There is little or no carryover from the bedroom to the rest of life. Lovers often take turns assuming sexual roles with each other.

Many gay men dispense with roles altogether, and do not connect fucking, say, with dominance, or sucking with passivity. To them, sensual pleasure is the main goal, and they do not attach much significance to who is doing what to whom. Still others enjoy deliberately playing a particular part.

Often these games are called scenes—captor/captive; delivery boy/house-holder; phone repairman/customer; ticketing policeman/driver; or examination giver/test taker. But they remain ready, willing, and able to swap roles midstream, thereby developing maximum flexibility in their role-playing repertoire (see *Bottom; Top; Types*).

Pornography is also a good outlet for various sorts of role-playing, or at least for experiencing role-playing fantasies.

SADOMASOCHISM

Sadomasochism is a sexual variation that celebrates virility, ritual, and pain. Its proponents adhere to sharply defined roles based upon power: master and slave, or "top man" and "bottom man." The word "sadomasochism" itself is derived from the name of two men: the Marquis de Sade and Leopold von Sacher-Masoch. De Sade (1740–1814) believed that pain, not pleasure, was the highest form of sexual activity. His *120 Days of Sodom* is filled with examples. Von Sacher-Masoch (1836–1895) was a historian and novelist. All his novels contained whipping scenes, and he himself preferred to be whipped by women wearing furs, especially if the women were older.

Many examples of sadomasochism can be drawn, curiously enough, from the history of the Catholic church. The flagellants, for instance, were a twelfth-century mass movement that encouraged people to flog themselves until the blood flowed. The lives of the saints are also replete with instances of masochism. In 1920, Saint Margaret Mary Alacoque was canonized. A seventeenth-century nun, she carved the name of Jesus on her chest with a knife, but because it didn't last long enough, she then burnt it in with a candle. At least as bizarre was Saint Mary-Magdalen dei Pazzi, who used to roll in thornbushes in the convent garden, then go into the convent and whip herself. She also forced novices to tie her to a post, insult her, whip her, and drop hot wax on her.

Although many gay men have dismissed S/M at one time or another, a large segment of the gay population continues to walk the streets of the cities garbed in black leather and chains or in uniforms such as those of motorcycle cops or marine MPs. Some men pull this off superbly. A guy with long straight hair slicked back with oil, a three-day growth of beard, a torn T-shirt, and muscled biceps, wearing leather chaps and motorcycle boots, can attract a lot of attention.

There is no simple explanation for the increased popularity of S/M, nor of its attractions. We offer as possibilities the following: First, this phenomenon is not confined to gay circles. We live in an era that glamorizes tough guys; many of the top stars at the box office are he-men. This is the popular image of male sex appeal. Second, not all the men in leather bars are actually sadomasochists; for some, denim and leather are just a fashion. Many

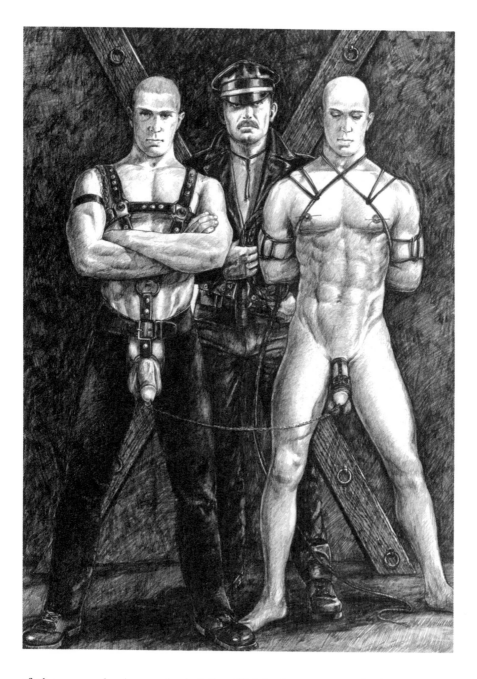

of the men who have adopted the S/M look are not really interested in inflicting pain or suffering it.

Sadomasochism has been around a long time; permissiveness has merely allowed it to appear more openly; desires that were always there, but hidden, are now paraded. Then, too, men in their forties and fifties have found acceptance in leather bars. The leather look can give strong allure to a man who has lost the charms of youth.

Our culture is a hierarchy of power, but in everyday life, power is clothed, not naked; hypocritical, not honest. Parents dominate children, men dominate women, whites dominate blacks, the rich dominate the poor, the boss dominates his employees, straights dominate gays. S/M dramatizes these situations and even temporarily reverses them, so the oppressed accountant by day becomes the oppressing sadist by night.

And tricking within the context of sadomasochism has certain advantages. So many of the attitudes, verbal exchanges, and sexual moves are ritualized and safely predictable that a one-night stand often lacks the fumbling and uncertainty that can characterize tricking in other contexts.

Finally, S/M can touch deep emotional chords. It may seem rigid, but it allows people to explore fantasies of domination and surrender, of cruelty and tenderness, of contempt and adoration.

Before getting involved in this scene, be aware that there are men for whom real violence is not only exciting, but essential. Occasionally, genuinely harmful things do happen. If you've decided to try the scene, start out with someone you know. You may be too naive to spot a potentially dangerous person (See *Cruising; Dangerous Sex*).

The novice often starts as a masochist. There's no way you can learn to be a good S except from someone experienced. Don't be too worried; the experienced S will let the novice establish his own limits. It's probably also a good idea to agree on a *safe word,* a signal that lets the S know that those limits have been reached. If you're with someone who refuses to use a safe word, don't get involved.

Another word about signals. Keys hung on the left and handkerchiefs in the left back pocket mark the sadist or "top man"; keys or handkerchiefs on the right indicate that the wearer is a masochist or "bottom man." Many men wear the insignia of motorcycle clubs, especially on the backs of denim jackets. They have no sexual significance except for the one showing two semicircles, one above another, each penetrated by a sharp line; this is the badge of the Fistfuckers of America (see *Fisting*). Some men into S/M are also into fisting. The Hell Fire Club is a group of men into serious S/M. It operates by invitation only and holds a yearly meeting, called Inferno, in the Midwest. The club's name is probably borrowed from the Hell-Fire Club organized by Sir Francis Dashwood in late eighteenth-century England.

The S/M scene tends to include the heavy use of drugs, since they help lower inhibitions and heighten fantasies.

Some S/M lovers who have been together for a long time maintain a strict role division. Usually, they do not carry this role-playing into ordinary life: The slave does not serve the master except during sex; otherwise he is equal. Other lovers who are into S/M reverse roles. Still others drift into ordinary gay sex with each other but play out S/M fantasies with strangers. (Read *S and M: Studies in Sadomasochism* by Weinberg and Karmel.)

The dividing line between S/M and other styles of sex play isn't always clear. Most men enjoy some roughness in their sex play from time to time.

A well-placed slap on the ass at the right time, or lots of dirty talk, can add extra excitement to an ordinary encounter. Tit clamps, dildos, ropes, and other toys can also be used to increase excitement (see *Bondage; Fisting; Nibbling and Biting; Nipples; Piercing; Sex Toys; Spanking; Vanilla*).

SAFE SEX

It's late at night, and you are partying with a friend at the most popular club in town. Perhaps you're at a gay summer resort like Fire Island in New York, or Fort Lauderdale in Florida, and men are dancing all around you. Many are in bathing suits or shorts, and the shared energy is intoxicating. As you whirl about the dance floor, you notice someone you spied on the beach earlier, a man you think is very sexy. You observe how he snaps his head back as he dances, trying to keep the hair out of his face, and how it just bounces back again. You wish you were assertive enough to walk over and while looking into his eyes, brush his hair back. You imagine yourself cupping his face in your hands, delicately kissing and caressing him. But you're too shy, and you tell yourself that someone as attractive as he is wouldn't be interested in you.

Only minutes later the unbelievable happens: Standing outside for a bit of fresh air with your dance partner, you hear someone say hello. The voice comes from behind. You turn around. "My name is Paul," he says, as he brushes his hair back. This gesture is enough to turn you on, and you blush. You're already getting hard. Your friend, diplomatically, makes himself scarce. You hardly know what you're saying as you and Paul chat together, and his words seem to float in the air, but never get into your ears. If you could only hear what he's saying.

An hour later, you're holding hands, back at a nearby cottage he's rented. Only the briefest moments are spent on the couch, and soon you two are lying together on the bed, kissing, caressing—and tasting one another. Then he turns on his back, spreads his legs and says, "Fuck me." He hands you a lubricant. You ask for a condom and he says, "I trust you." You've gone to bed with a fool. A cute fool, maybe, but also a deadly one.

The scenario might be different. Paul might want to fuck you. Again, no condom. He might say, "You're the only person I've ever fucked without a rubber." In this case he's not a fool; he's a liar. You're the fool if you believe him.

Why do men endanger their lives by having unsafe sex? First, our impression is that it is the younger, rather than the older, men who are violating safe-sex guidelines, believing "it can't happen to me." Other young men feel deprived, contrary, and rebellious. One youth said, "You guys [meaning the older generation of gay men] had all the fun! You got to do everything. And what are we stuck with? Rubbers and hand jobs?"

A second reason is that men are turned on by visual stimuli, by seeing an attractive face and body. It stimulates all the sexual hormones in the body, and as the Yiddish proverb says, "When the prick is hard, the brains are soft!" Imagine, then, how difficult restraint is when visual and tactile senses are being overstimulated by so many apparently available men in a club or at a bar. We also know that using alcohol and drugs interferes with good judgment (see *Booze and Highs*). As one psychologist noted, "The superego is soluble in alcohol." Then, too, some men fear offending a potential sex partner by insisting on safe sex, especially if that partner is physically desirable (see *Saying No*), while others are unable to fight peer pressure: If "everyone else is doing it," so will they, even if it kills them.

All these factors may explain why some men appear to go into something like a fugue state (psychologists call it "denial"), a sort of amnesia, forgetting friends and lovers who are ill or dead.

Making choices about sex is very important now that HIV Disease is so much a part of our lives. Most of us have seen close friends, lovers, and other family members die. It is crucial that all of us understand the parameters of safe sex, not only to protect our own health, but also to maintain the health of our community.

Being in love can lead to life-threatening mistakes, especially for men who have come out during the AIDS epidemic. Newcomers to the gay world bring with them a reservoir of love. For the first time in their lives they can express their romantic feelings as they search for lovers. Some gay men act as though they're more terrified of being abandoned by a potential lover than they are of the transmission of the HIV virus. They have unsafe sex with someone they love, rationalizing, "I'm afraid he'll think I don't love him," or, "He'll leave me if I tell him I don't want to take his come," jeopardizing both their and their lover's lives. A friend might reply, "Schmuck, how much can he love you if he's willing to put your life in danger?"

Many gay men behave as though safe sex guidelines didn't exist. It's not because these men are stupid or lack information. The guidelines are fairly easy to understand. You'll find them listed at the end of this section. Most gay magazines and every AIDS organization publishes the latest information about safe sex.

Your sexual behavior is an expression of how you feel about yourself. If you respect yourself, safe sex won't be a problem. Sexual behavior is also an expression of your feelings about other men. When you cajole, exploit, or manipulate someone in bed, you're not expressing sexual needs. Your lust is a cover-up. Perhaps you're angry at all men, or you're resentful over an unresolved childhood incident or a disappointment in a previous love affair. All these can be motivations for exploiting another.

Gay men have three responsibilities with respect to safe sex. The first is to oneself. If you have self-respect, you won't do anything to put your own life in danger. Your second responsibility is to others. You should do whatever you can to influence the sexual behavior of your friends, tricks, and potential lovers. Tell them you want them to have a good sex life; you just don't want them to die. Teach them about safe sex, and show them where to get more information.

Your third responsibility is to the gay community. We hope you'll join the struggle of other gay men and lesbians to pressure our government to find a cure for AIDS. If you can, join ACT UP or Queer Nation, or serve as a volunteer in an AIDS organization. Keep in mind that the only way gay people have secured our rights is by demanding them. As a gay man in a gay community, your example is an important part of that struggle (see *Booze and Highs; Gay Liberation; Saying No*).

Considered Safe

Mutual masturbation
Hugging
Body rubbing
Massage
Dry kissing
S/M if without bleeding or bruising
Sex toys used only on yourself

Considered Possibly Safe

Anal intercourse with a condom
Wet kissing
Sucking, but stopping before climax
External water sports (no swallowing)

Considered Unsafe

Swallowing semen
Anal intercourse without a condom
Water sports in mouth or on skin with sores
Sharing IV needles
Sharing enema equipment or sex toys
Fisting
Rimming

SAYING NO

Many men are so afraid of offending other people that it is only with great difficulty that they can say no to invitations. This inability can lead to touchy situations, particularly when the invitation is sexual.

Directness is always best when you're saying no. Lengthy and complicated excuses rarely work; they tend to get taken at face value, and often all you achieve is deferral of the invitation. Softening a negative response with smiles, shrugs, and equivocations—"That's a really nice invitation, but I don't think I really should, at least not this time, I guess"—is ineffective. The equivocation betrays uncertainty on your part and invites renewed appeals from the other person. He pressures you, and more often than not, you give in.

There's only one solution; take a deep breath and, politely but with no trace of hesitation, say no. A firm "No, thank you" to a sexual invitation is much kinder than an unnecessarily rude response, or no response at all. He may not be your cup of tea but he's still a person with feelings, and he dislikes being rejected as much as you do.

The AIDS epidemic has added a new dimension to saying no. We are now forced to say no to men who excite us sexually, but who won't respect safe sex guidelines. These men should be avoided even though they may stir the greatest passion in us. One needn't say no to another man who's seropositive or who has HIV Disease, because you can protect each other from transmitting the virus (see *Body Fluids; Body Positive; Safe Sex*). But someone who acts as if there *isn't* an epidemic is himself ensuring its continuation. If you still feel such a man is hot, go home and jerk off while fantasizing about having sex with him. Whatever you do, don't take him with you.

SCAT

A small minority of gay men like to make feces a part of the sex scene. The word for this—"scat"—is derived from the Greek word for dung, which is the root of "scatology," meaning the study of filth or obscenity. Scat is probably more talked about than performed.

Some guys who are into scat shit on each other or eat each other's shit or smear it over their bodies. For others, it's not the physical aspect of shit so much as its symbolic value that counts. Rather than using shit to degrade themselves and each other, they use it in a variety of metaphoric, even ritualistic ways, often without touching it: experiencing it being produced by another; sometimes adoring it (in almost the same way that infants play with it as a marvelous product of their own body); stuffing it into condoms and using it as a substitute penis.

Scat may be associated with S/M, although not necessarily so. A few leather guys indulge in this scene; in an S/M context the master shits on his slave as yet another way to humiliate and degrade him. Among masochists in search of extremes, scat must represent the ultimate indignity—and therefore the ultimate turn-on. There is no reason to believe that someone who eats shit during sex invites or tolerates humiliation in his everyday life. "Scat" merely describes a sexual act, not a social role.

Scat, like rimming, does of course expose you to hepatitis, a variety of parasites, and bacillary dysentery (see *HIV Disease; Rimming; Sexually Transmitted Diseases*).

The scat scene is a curious one for psychologists. They have no idea how it originates, although they assume that some psychological trauma in childhood causes feces to become eroticized. By the average person, scat is considered kinky, and by the professional, as one of the paraphilias (see *Dangerous Sex*).

SEDUCTION

The term has come to have such a negative connotation—enticing a novice so as to have your wicked way with him—that we sometimes forget that seduction can be an exciting game for both the seducer and the seduced.

Right from the beginning, you have to make a choice whether to go for immediate sex or to attempt an affair (see *Cruising*). Each requires slight modifications in seduction technique. Affairs usually start with courtship. Even if you meet in a bar in an obvious pickup situation, you might ask for his phone number rather than going home with him that very night and having sex; instant sex may cut the tension between you and allow you to fall into a wham-bam-thank-you-Sam cycle. Far better, if you have serious intentions, is to phone him the next day and invite him to dinner or a movie, perhaps on a prime-time weekend evening. He may be puzzled by your wanting to put off sex, but he may also be intrigued and complimented.

On your date, ask all about him and speak freely about yourself in return. Don't stress your weaknesses and shortcomings. Later on, if you become close, you can share misgivings about yourself and talk about your problems.

Don't discuss the casual sex you've had, though you might feel free to mention love affairs. The note to sound is intimate, not chummy; romantic, not social. Engage his interests and address yourself to his hopes and anxieties. Most men in their twenties, for instance, are as much concerned with their careers as with finding a lover. Make yourself doubly attractive by giving him a chance to discuss these aspirations.

If a one-night stand is your aim, the approach will be different. As soon as you meet someone at a party or club, make your intention clear by moving the conversation toward the topic of sex. Many men are offended if you ask exactly what they like to do in bed; they prefer to let things take their course without prior discussion. Keep the conversation flirty, filled with innuendo, and pay him several discreet sexual compliments. The aim is to create an erotic tension in which you two are the only people who

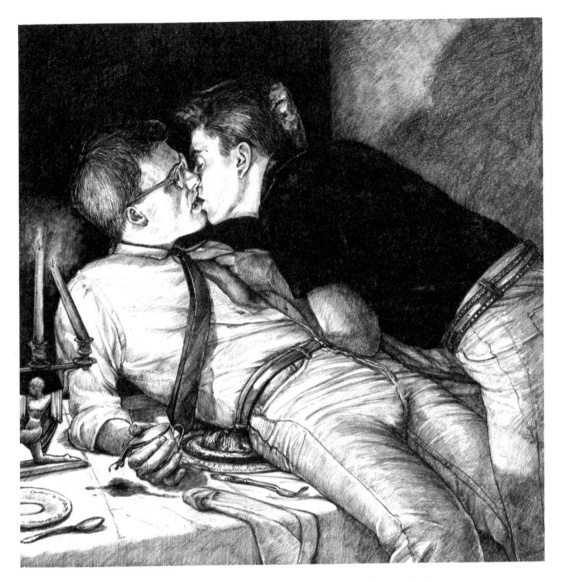

count, a tension that can only be resolved through sex. Before sex you should do nothing to destroy the fantasy you're carefully weaving about the two of you.

Some men have gone a step further in their seduction technique. All they have to do is get the man home, where they've exercised their erotic imagination in designing an atmosphere so seductive no one can resist. The lights are all on rheostats; a stereo bathes the room in sound. The bed is low, immense, and covered with bolsters; the rug soft and inviting should sex spill over onto the floor; the windows curtained for privacy, the room relatively soundproof. Some bedrooms are so designed that a flick of a switch dims the lights and starts a porno video (see *Pornography*). Other men think such a bedroom too contrived for their tastes. Perhaps the best advice is to develop a good sense of humor, a bit of style, and lots of charm. With these traits, in the right proportions, men will be drawn to you like iron to a magnet.

SEX ADS

Sexual advertisements can be found in gay newspapers and magazines as well as in "alternative" newspapers, where they begin "GWM," meaning "gay white male," or "GBM," meaning "gay black male." Because personal ads are costly and outline specific requirements, an entire shorthand has developed, which can provide fairly detailed information. Here is an ad taken from a newspaper:

> MASCULINE
>
> 23 W Bott BB 6'3" br/bl vgdlkg HIV − 185# 7½" cut Fr A/P Gr P. Seeks prof. big Lat/Medit top hung uncut dom kinky 30s-40s HIV −. All photo/phones get replies. Box XYZ, Anywhere, CA.

Let's decode this. We discover that the man putting the ad into the magazine begins by describing himself. He is "masculine," which means butch or straight-looking.

Next, he's twenty-three years old, white-skinned, a bottom (see *Bottom*), a bodybuilder. He then gives his height, his hair color (brown) the color of his eyes (blue), and (immodestly) adds that he is *very* good-looking. He then notes his HIV antibody status, his weight, and the length of his cock, adding that he is circumcised (cut). Finally he lists the sexual activities he prefers: "Fr A/P"—"French active or passive"—means he will suck cock and get sucked. "Greek passive" means he will get fucked but doesn't wish to fuck anyone else.

The next sentence in the ad begins with the word "Seeks" and details the kind of man the advertiser's looking for: a big man, preferably of Latino or Mediterranean background. A top man (see *Top*), hung (i.e., with a big dick), uncircumcised. He adds that he'd like the man he's seeking to be dominant and kinky. Furthermore, he specifies the age of his preferred partner—somewhat older than himself—and the preferred HIV antibody status. The final sentence tells the reader that if he sends a photograph of himself and includes his phone number, the advertiser will reply without fail. He finishes with his post-office box number, city, and zip code.

Here's another ad from the same issue of the same newspaper.

> COUNTRY MAN
>
> Seeks same for friendship or more. Interested in farm or outdoor worker. I am 38 5'11" 155#, gr/br. Will travel, NY, PA. Reply to Box #123, Syracuse NY area.

This ad needs little in the way of explanation. The man is saying he has a simple life, simple needs, and simple requirements. He's less concerned with anything specifically physical or even sexual in a partner than in sharing a particular kind of life and interests. Travel is emphasized because gay men are so spread out in rural areas.

Obviously, ads can be as detailed or as vague, as friendly or as aloof, as professional or as giddily romantic as you want them to be. You write them; you answer them: You're the boss!

When should you advertise for sex or romance? When you have spare money and are feeling somewhat open, even experimental—after all, you'll be meeting new people, so get ready for new experiences. If you have very specific sexual needs and requirements, you may *have* to advertise to find someone in your area who shares these tastes.

When should you answer a sex ad? When you're a little bored with the same old people and things in your life. Some guys have had amazing luck placing and answering ads; others have had no luck at all. There's only one way to find out which category you fit into.

It's generally a good idea to talk on the phone with your potential sex partner until you feel comfortable. Feel free to discuss all and any issues— safety, health, HIV status—then meet with him. If you're *still* not sure about him or nervous, meet him in a neutral or public place. If you meet and you don't like his looks or otherwise feel the date is not going to work out, either tell him outright or, if you can't be so blatant, try to steer your discussion off sexual topics and onto more general ones. After all, there's no reason why you can't have a friendly chat.

SEX CLUBS

During the 1980s, as the gay community became aware that the HIV virus was being transmitted among gay men in bathhouses, most of the baths were closed (see *Baths*). But gay men have always looked for private, enclosed sanctuaries of relative safety where they can meet other men for sex. Jerk-off clubs were, and still are, the primary replacement for baths and back rooms (see *J.O. Clubs*)—they are private, popular, and safe.

In the last few years, however, a new institution has arisen in a few large cities—the sex club. Whereas the jerk-off club discourages sucking and fucking, the sex club tacitly encourages them by providing an anything-goes orgy atmosphere reminiscent of the wildest days of the baths.

We have visited a few of these clubs and found them to be extraordinarily *unsafe* environments in which to have sex. They may even be a major factor in the "second wave" of new HIV infection showing up in the gay community. In these clubs, a number of men, particularly younger men, are allowing themselves to be fucked without a condom—a foolish, self-destructive act—while the men fucking them seem to not care that by gratifying their own needs they are perpetuating the AIDS epidemic.

We unconditionally discourage participation in sex clubs because they are unsafe environments (see *Safe Sex*).

SEX TOYS

Sex boutiques sell a wide range of merchandise. Among the items most commonly offered for sale is an enormous range of aids for curing sexual dysfunctions: creams to delay ejaculation; machines and salves to cure impotence; and aphrodisiacs to enhance sexual desire. They are all expensive, useless junk. However, regarded as amusements and not cures, sex toys can add variety and excitement to your erotic life. You can insert your cock into a rubber or plastic sheath, and a partial vacuum that builds and releases on the principle of a cow milker will suck you off. A more expensive model will suck and fuck you at the same time, or suck you and your partner simultaneously. Electric vibrators slipped over the back of the hand can introduce novelty into masturbation. There are battery-operated vibrators in the shape of cocks, which you can use to fuck yourself.

There are *dildos* in all sizes, some eight inches in circumference, others nearly a yard long. Don't use one longer than ten inches, or you may damage yourself. Perhaps you should start with a small one and get used to it. While you can't trade them in like used cars, dildos are inexpensive. The dildo should be made of soft, flexible material, either rubber or pliant plastic. Hard plastic or metal dildos are dangerous, as are those that can be cranked and twisted about in your ass (a metal wire runs down the center of the tube and might poke out and puncture the wall of the rectum). Be sure the dildo has balls or a wide base so it can't slip up your ass beyond the point of retrieval, which might require surgery. A double dildo (called a double dong) is a long rubber tube with a glans at either end. Some couples coordinate their movements while using it, so that each partner gets fucked simultaneously. *Remember, don't put candles, bottles, light bulbs, or any other objects up your ass—and don't let anyone else do it to you* (see *Dangerous Sex; Saying No*).

An entire class of sex toys consists of gadgets associated with S/M, such as chains, belts, handcuffs, whips, nightsticks, and other instruments of authority and punishment. Others were first associated with S/M but have now become ubiquitous in the gay scene. *Cock rings* are devices placed around the bottom of the penis and the balls while the cock is soft or semihard. After the cock becomes fully hard, the ring cuts off the outflow of blood and prolongs the erection. There are several kinds of cock rings: metal loops of varying size, leather straps that snap shut, and leather thongs that are tied around the cock and balls. The leather strap is the most comfortable and the easiest to get on and off, but many men prefer the hardness (and coldness) of thick metal rings. Mind you, many metal rings are thick enough to set off metal detectors. This can lead to embarrassing (or hysterically funny) situations in airports as you try to explain to the authorities why you keep setting off the security alarms.

Another device often sold as a sex aid but much more useful as a sex toy is the *cock-enlargement pump*. Most of these consist of a plastic tube (into which you insert your cock) and a pump attachment. We've recently noticed that some J.O. clubs have sponsored "Pump Nights" for those into vacuum pumps. Essentially the pump is a device for masturbation. It will certainly not enlarge your cock, no matter what the ads promise. *Always be careful when using this device!* The cock has a rich and sensitive vascular system; abusing it can damage blood vessels. Manual machines are preferable to automatic pumps, which could get out of control.

Tit clamps are very popular. These metal clips, sometimes lined with rubber, boost sensation when placed on the nipples. They can also cause excruciating pain. Snakebite kits have rubber sucking cups that serve the same purpose. *Tit rings* are inserted through pierced nipples, just as earrings are placed through the earlobe. They are less painful to wear than tit clamps (see *Piercing*). Sometimes a leather thong or metal chain is strung through the tit rings and given to the sadist to play with. Many masochists enjoy tit action during sex, especially when they are sucking off their master.

Sometimes weights are attached to a slave's balls. As he becomes more aroused, heavier weights are added. Other, more exotic gear includes leather or latex masks, gags, dog collars, and leashes. Male "chastity belts" are also available. They consist of a leather belt around the waist, a strong snap that goes between the legs, and a dildo inserted up the ass and held in place by the strap. Some of those trim executives you see dashing about town or presiding over committee meetings are sitting on a six-inch dildo only their masters can remove. Less extreme, but also popular, is the *butt plug,* a rubber object shorter than a dildo that when inserted keeps the asshole from tightening up. Use one if you have a big-cocked lover who likes to fuck you often.

Ambitious sex boutiques may offer a great many more devices and toys, including such large S/M contraptions as racks, stockades, and slings. These are all for gays with large bank accounts.

Remember, sex toys *must* be cleaned after use. In most cases washing them well with hot, soapy water will do. However, if there's any doubt, or if the skin of anyone in the scene has been broken, do the following: Wash the toy with soap and water, then thoroughly rub it with alcohol. Finally, give it a second wash to get the alcohol off. This procedure ensures not only your own health, but the health of future sex partners.

SEX WITH ANIMALS

Sex with animals seems to have been quite common, although it was punished harshly in the Western world. It was labeled sodomy by both the church and the courts, a category that also included masturbation, anal intercourse, oral-genital contact, and *coitus interruptus* (pulling out before you come). For example, in 1642, Thomas Granger, a teenager who lived in Plymouth Colony, confessed to and was found guilty of buggery with a mare, a cow, two goats, five sheep, two calves, and a turkey. Now that's what you call a sexual appetite! The sex historian Vern Bullough tells us: "Though there was some difficulty in identifying the sheep so unnaturally used, mixed as they were with the flock, somehow five were selected to be executed along with the other animals, and they were burned in a great pit." Young Granger himself was also executed.

The Chinese were constantly accused of having "love affairs with geese." Both Sir Richard Burton (the English explorer) and Paolo Mantegazza (an Italian anthropologist) accused them of fucking geese and wringing the necks of the animals at the moment of ejaculation so as to "get the pleasurable benefit of the anal sphincter's last spasms in the victim." French farmers were said to do the same; they claimed to have learned the sex practice from the English. And sex with animals is probably the only thing never blamed on the Italians.

One supposes life on the average farm was lonely much of the time. Shepherds tending their flocks day after boring day must have done a certain amount of jerking off in the fields. No surprise if, over time, they started fucking sheep. Only the most sexually repressed would blame them, though admittedly we city boys snicker about farm boys fucking the livestock.

There doesn't seem to be a lot of sex with animals these days, although perhaps it's merely closeted. We suspect the incidence of animal sex is lower than it's ever been because of so much mechanization on the farm, the population shift to urban centers, and the replacement of family farms with corporate ones.

Moralists condemn sex with animals as disgusting, immoral, and generally horrible. Fortunately it's no longer a crime in a great many places, and nowhere in the United States is it a capital crime. We disagree with the moralists. Lots of children looked at and played with the genitals of their pet cats and dogs, and we've heard of more than one who has masturbated his pet dog. Like other inexperienced city dwellers, we may not so readily fathom the mechanics of cow-, sheep- or horse-fucking, but see no reason to condemn it out of hand. We hope it doesn't become the *only* sexual contact in a man's life.

Frederick the Great took a practical attitude. During an important battle, he observed a soldier he recognized, fettered in irons. "Why is that excellent soldier in irons?" he asked of the officer in charge. "For bestiality with his horse" was the reply." "Fool," said Frederick the Great, "don't put him in irons, put him in the infantry."

SEXUALLY TRANSMITTED DISEASES

lthough male homosexuals have been afflicted by venereal diseases for centuries, the medical profession has only recognized VD in gays in the past twenty-five years. Homophobic doctors have often refused to treat gay patients, or have viewed our health problems with such distaste that they in effect discouraged gay patients from seeking medical attention. This shoddy treatment made many gays, particularly those from small towns and rural areas, wary of physicians.

All gay men should have a basic knowledge of the sexually transmitted diseases, so they can recognize the symptoms in themselves and in their sexual partners. It then becomes the responsibility of each person to insist on being given the correct diagnostic tests and treatment by his physician (see *Finding a Physician*).

Sexually transmitted diseases (STD, for short) can be divided into two major categories. One comprises *venereal diseases*—those which directly affect the genitals. (The term "venereal" comes from Venus, the Roman goddess of love.) The primary venereal diseases are syphilis and gonorrhea, which are discussed below. The other major category comprises sexually transmitted diseases that do not directly affect the genitals. They are crabs, hepatitis, herpes, parasitic amoebas, prostatitis and urethritis, scabies, and venereal warts.

Gonorrhea

Gonorrhea, or "clap," is a major health problem in gays. About 15 percent of men who get gonorrhea in the penis *do not* develop symptoms, and even those who have symptoms may not develop them for two weeks. That makes detection difficult. Carriers without symptoms can transmit the disease without knowing it. Therefore, men who practice unsafe sex should have a routine VD checkup every six months (every three months if you're having sex with a lot of men), which means both a smear and urinalysis for clap and a blood test for syphilis. A blood test alone will not diagnose gonorrhea. Even if you do have regular checkups, remember that you can unwittingly infect an awful lot of people before you discover you have clap.

The slang term "clap" probably comes from "Mother Clap," whose real name was Margaret Clap. She ran a bawdyhouse for homosexual men in Holborn, a section of London. Thirty to forty men a night were entertained there until one day in 1726, when she was charged with keeping a "sodomitical house." The poor lady was fined, pilloried, and sentenced to two years.

You can get clap in the cock by fucking someone without a rubber or by getting a blow job from someone whose mouth is infected. Clap is caused by bacteria that invade the cells of the urethra (the canal that carries urine). If treatment is delayed, infection will spread throughout the urethra. Symptoms normally appear any time between twenty-four hours and five days after exposure. The chief symptoms are a discharge of a thick, creamy pus, and burning during urination. By milking down your cock you can see the earliest signs of pus. You should also check your underwear; the dried pus will make the pouch of your underwear stiff.

If you get fucked by someone without a rubber, you may develop clap in the ass. Symptoms are usually slower to show up in the rectum (if they develop at all) and detection is certain only by either looking at a smear under a microscope or culturing the germ in a laboratory. If your physician is not gay or is not used to treating gay patients, tell him the treatment for gonorrhea is Ceftriaxone. The symptoms you might notice are rectal fullness (feeling as if you have to defecate), pain, frequent farting, rectal bleeding, hemorrhoids, pus or blood in the stool, diarrhea, constipation, and sometimes an inability to piss. This urinary retention is brought about when bladder nerves are infected by gonorrhea. (These symptoms don't necessarily mean you have gonorrhea. Only a test can determine this.)

If your doctor is heterosexual or is unfamiliar with gay health problems, do not let him catheterize you (stick a tube up your penis to induce urination). Suggest that he test you for gonorrhea in the rectum; if you have it, then you should be given a shot of Ceftriaxone. Soon you will be able to piss again, though at first it might help to take a warm bath and try to piss in the hot water. Don't be reticent about asking for an anal smear. Some straight physicians are shy about asking if you need one, and you will have to direct such a doctor to do it.

Gay men also contract gonorrhea in the throat by sucking cock. Symptoms are often absent, but when present are a sore throat, a cough, upper respiratory congestion, and other coldlike disturbances. Sometimes the glands under the jaw swell up. Clap in the throat is less frequent than clap in the penis and anus, but then again it depends upon your sexual behavior.

You cannot get clap from kissing or from contact with toilet seats, towels, or cups; the bacteria need a constant supply of carbon dioxide, and die seconds after they are exposed to the air.

Gonorrhea should always be treated immediately. If it is not, the acute symptoms will go away after about six months, but the disease may lead to arthritis, pericarditis (inflammation of the sac around the heart), or emphysema.

All these suggestions, of course, must be confirmed by your physician. He alone can prescribe treatment, though you should insist that he take a "cure culture" after treatment. That means testing you again for the disease.

Syphilis

Syphilis is less common than gonorrhea, but it's more serious and must be carefully monitored. If you are sexually active you should receive a blood test at least every six months.

The first outbreak of the disease appeared in 1494 among French soldiers stationed in Naples. The Italians called it the French disease, while the French called it the Neapolitan disease. When it arrived in Turkey, the Turks called it the Christian disease. And the Chinese called it the Portuguese disease. Everyone finally agreed to blame it on Columbus and the Native Americans.

The first symptom of syphilis is a red sore called a *chancre* (about the size of a pea), though this sore does not always appear. The skin breaks open to reveal the chancre, which may soon be covered by a yellow or gray scab. It is painless and does not bleed easily. It may appear on your penis, in your mouth, or in your anus. Left untreated, the chancre heals by itself in a few weeks; unfortunately, the disease continues to develop.

The sore, if it appears, can show up ten days after sexual contact but ordinarily occurs about three weeks after infection. Aside from it there are no symptoms, except that lymph nodes often become tender, inflamed, and enlarged to the size of grapes.

Secondary syphilis starts about four to six weeks after the initial infection. A rash, which does not necessarily itch, breaks out (usually all over the body); it can appear even on the palms and the soles of the feet. The patient has a general feeling of ill health—headaches, nausea, loss of appetite, and fever. The hair sometimes falls out. (Luckily it grows back.) In the secondary stage the individual is highly contagious: he can transmit syphilis through all the mucous membranes, including those of the mouth and anus. This second set of symptoms will also disappear within a few weeks, but then the illness enters a third, even more dangerous stage.

For several years the untreated disease will be latent in the body. There will probably be no symptoms, though a sore may appear on the site of the original infection after a year or two. Once a year has passed (though it does take a year), the patient is no longer infectious. Some advanced cases will move on to tertiary syphilis. There are three kinds: One, benign, is characterized by the development of large lesions in and on the body, the second, *cardiovascular syphilis,* often ends in death from heart failure. The third kind, *paresis,* leads to the deterioration of the central nervous system and psychosis. This stage is usually reached ten to twenty years after the initial infection.

Syphilis can be cured easily if caught in its early stages. However, the presence of HIV infection complicates the treatment of syphilis (see *HIV Disease*). The blood test for syphilis is usually negative during the first four or five weeks of the infection, but then it turns positive. Blood tests are not always reliable for early syphilis infection, so if you have disturbing symptoms have a second test even if the results of the first were negative. The treatment for early syphilis is a large dose of penicillin, though other antibiotics are used for people allergic to this drug. And don't forget that follow-up blood test.

Crabs

These little devils are lice that are often picked up during sex. They are relatively harmless, though they itch like hell. They grow chiefly in the pubic hair but may also be found under the arms, on the chest, around the crotch, and between the buttocks. They can cling to hairs on the legs all the way down to the knees and have sometimes been found on hairy forearms and even in the eyebrows or beard.

You can see crabs if you look hard enough. They are dark in color and usually live at the base of the hair follicle. You may also notice little blood spots on your underwear.

The best treatments are liquid preparations called A-200 and Rid, which can be bought in drugstores without a prescription. Your physician, however, may want to prescribe Kwell. All medications come with careful instructions regarding their use. Remove all your clothing before putting on the A-200 or Kwell; shower afterward; then launder your towels, sheets, jeans, and underwear. Be sure to tell all your sexual partners to treat themselves for crabs, or you'll be reinfecting each other for months.

Hepatitis

This serious liver disease is widespread in the gay community. It is communicated in many ways—by kissing, by contact with any of the mucous membranes, by eating infected shellfish, by rimming (fecal–oral transmission), by infected semen (introduced orally or anally), and through transfusions of infected blood. There are at least three types of hepatitis: "infectious" (now called *Type A*); "serum" (*Type B*); and *Type C,* which is similar to Type B. Symptomatically, they are all similar.

The early signs resemble the symptoms of flu—muscle aches and pains, fatigue, and intermittent fever. Sometimes a rash breaks out as well. Soon these symptoms disappear and you become extremely fatigued. Your urine turns mahogany brown and your shit becomes gray-white. Smokers lose their taste for cigarettes. Nausea and nearly complete loss of appetite occur; then your eyeballs and skin turn yellow (this is called *jaundice*). By this time, the worst is over, though you certainly won't look your best.

There is no cure for hepatitis, just supportive treatment. You must be under your doctor's care. He may suggest you rest whenever your body says you need sleep, eat a bland diet, and during the acute stage eliminate all fats (otherwise you'll be nauseated). *Cut out liquor and recreational drugs for at least six months after you regain your health.* Take a multiple vitamin daily. In the past, complete bed rest was recommended during the acute stage, but there is now evidence that moderate exercise is preferable. You will not be able to work for at least two weeks, however, and during this period you will sleep more hours than you're awake. Only in exceptionally severe cases is there reason to be hospitalized; home care is normally quite adequate. Your roommate or a friend will have to run errands for you.

If you have been exposed to hepatitis, your doctor may want to give you a shot of gamma globulin. The incubation period for hepatitis is two or three weeks for Type A and three weeks to ninety days for Type B. There is now an effective vaccine for hepatitis B.

You can get hepatitis more than once, and a relapse is also possible. It is a very serious disease. About 1 percent of the people who get hepatitis will die from it.

Herpes

These viral infections are caused by the same virus that causes cold sores; they are usually seen on the penis, especially just under the foreskin, though they can show up anywhere on the body, including the face. They can be transmitted during sex. During sexual intercourse they often make fucking painful.

There is no cure for herpes. The disease goes away unpredictably on its own, though it can reappear, especially during stress.

Parasites

The gay community has been heavily hit by sexually transmitted parasites, which cause gastrointestinal health problems. Doctors should check gay patients routinely for parasites, especially if the patients have bowel complaints.

There are two kinds of parasites that have become common among gays (and many straights): *Entamoeba histolytica* and *Giardia lamblia*. Many people who travel to foreign destinations return home with these pests, which entered their bodies through contaminated food and water. Both varieties produce similar symptoms, which can range from no outward signs at all to violent dysentery. In between these extremes are such symptoms as soft stools, abdominal cramps, unusually smelly stools, gas, fatigue, fever and chills, loss of appetite, nausea, and sometimes vomiting. Parasites produce a general malaise.

Parasites are also anally–orally transmitted. That is, if you rim someone you run a high risk of getting them. Don't be too confident that you're safe even if you never rim people, because there are many intermediate and hard-to-discern methods of transmission: For instance, sucking someone's cock during anonymous sex. Your partner may have been fucking someone with parasites just before he met you. Someone who has not washed his hands after shitting may prepare a salad for you and transmit parasites in that way. Hands are frequent carriers of parasites.

Diagnosis is difficult unless you go to a trained parasitologist or unless your doctor works with a lab technician who knows what to look for. Tropical-disease centers are particularly knowledgeable about parasites. Usually a test is made upon a bit of fecal matter. The parasitologist can simply extract a bit of feces from the anus with a Q-tip, put it on a slide, and examine it under the microscope. A wet stool test, however, is sometimes necessary in hard-to-detect cases. There are effective medications to rid the body of parasites. Treatment lasts from a couple of weeks to a few months.

Prostatitis and Urethritis

Prostatitis is an infection of the prostate gland. Prostatitis is not a problem that is sexually transmitted, strictly speaking, but sometimes bacteria that enter the urethral canal during anal sex can work their way into the prostate and cause infection. Symptoms of prostatitis are burning in the urethra during urination and more frequent urination than usual. An erection is not painful, but sometimes ejaculation hurts. Pain is occasionally felt in or behind the testicles, and once in a while specks of blood show up in the semen or urine. Inflammation of the prostate can be a side effect of penile gonorrhea. A more frequent cause, however, is occasional bursts of sexual activity followed by irregular periods of inactivity. Yet another cause is delayed ejaculation. If you have an enlarged prostate, your doctor may recommend that you not get fucked until the swelling is reduced.

The major cause of nongonococcal urethritis is *chlamydia*. Chlamydia is fast becoming the number one STD in heterosexuals, and so it can be spread to those gays who have sex with straight men. In general, it's far less common in the gay population. About 60 percent of all the cases of an inflamed urethral canal are called *nonspecific urethritis* (NSU) but may be caused by chlamydia. The primary symptoms of this very contagious condition are burning of the urethra during urination, and a discharge (usually clear). Vigorous sexual activity can also cause abrasion of the penis that may lead to urethritis. Perfumed soaps and bubble baths can also cause urethral irritations. If you have a discharge of any sort, see your doctor and alert your partner.

While chlamydia is treatable, nonspecific urethritis is usually treated by refraining from sexual activity of all kinds for a period of a few days, by which time the condition has usually improved.

Scabies

Scabies are common among gay men. They are tiny parasites that live just below the surface of the skin, usually around the wrists, but often on the ankles, near the groin and under the arms. They are very itchy, especially at night. They are transmitted by skin contact, but they can also be picked up from sheets and towels. If not treated, they will not produce dangerous symptoms, but they are annoying. The preferred treatment is Kwell lotion, which must be prescribed by your doctor.

Venereal Warts

Venereal warts are caused by a virus, often transmitted during sex. You can develop a venereal wart on the rectum or on the penis.

The warts are not usually painful in themselves, but they can become irritated and make fucking uncomfortable. If you and a regular lover or partner both have warts, do not resume sex until you both have been cured, or the contagious nature of the warts will lead to continued reinfection. Lasers are now used to treat warts.

SHAVING

The sudden appearance of pubic and body hair, along with other changes accompanying puberty, such as the deepening of the voice and the surge of sexual desire, is surely the most dramatic event in the life of many boys. Yet paradoxically, because things like body hair quickly come to seem so natural, and sexual longings quickly become so all-encompassing in our imagination, it's often close to impossible for adult men to recall how their bodies looked and felt before they passed through the great hormonal divide.

Of all the changes that occur at puberty, only the presence of body hair is changeable. Maybe it's for this reason that some men like to recapture their boyishness by shaving their bodies.

The first thing you'll discover when you shave your crotch, your chest, your armpits, or your legs is a deliciously heightened sensitivity. Every inch of your newly mown skin will sing as thigh rubs thigh or pant leg, balls rub against underwear, or chest rubs against shirt. Your whole body will be much more sensitive against your sheets. The intensified sensation you'll experience might feel something like the focused, heightened awareness of bodily sensations some guys say so-called sex-enhancing drugs induce. But remember, as body hair begins to grow back, it will itch quite a lot. Only those with the most refined and peculiar sensibilities will enjoy that feeling for long.

Shaving your body will make your skin smoother and will tend to make you look more boyish, feminine, or androgynous. This is not everybody's idea of a good time, of course, but it will be a big turn-on to some. Admiring yourself in a mirror or stroking your smooth, shorn skin (or having your partner do it) may excite your sexual imagination and heighten masturbatory pleasure.

There are many reasons why a man might prefer a hairless partner. You might want to offer your lover a new thrill. You might want to attract a new type—men who prefer smooth boyish bodies. For other guys, a preference for smooth skin beneath them may simply be aesthetic or tied to unfathomable preconscious associations; Eros often leads us to prefer certain appearances and activities. So if you feel more fuckable with the kind of elegant legs that would look good in nylons, go ahead, enjoy the fantasy.

The actual mechanics of shaving are easy. If you are fairly limber, most of your body except your back is within reach. When you get to your balls you will have to make your wrinkled skin taut by holding onto the base of the sac and pulling the skin tight.

For many men, shaving—especially shaving the crotch area—has become a prelude to, even a part of sex with their partner. The act connotes trust, intimacy, and also a special bond between the men not available otherwise.

Allowing someone else to shave you, just your balls or your whole body, may bring you in touch with all sorts of little-boy fantasies (see *Daddy-Son Fantasies*). If you are going to be shaving someone else, remember you're likely to draw a little blood, and if there is any doubt in your mind about the health of the person you're playing with, wear medical gloves. It's also a good idea to have a bunch of disposable razors on hand. Don't forget there's a lot more surface area on the body than on the face, and on some hairy guys the skin is overgrown with a lush jungle. You don't want to run out of razors when half his crotch is shaved. As far as we know, asymmetrical or random-pattern shaving has not yet made it into fashionable gay consciousness. Don't use depilatories on or around your asshole because they burn like hell.

SIDE BY SIDE

This is a very comfortable and peaceful position for fucking. Both men lie on their sides, one with his back to the other (spoonlike). The man behind lubricates a finger and opens up his partner's asshole with patience and tenderness. When the muscles are fully relaxed, he slowly pushes his cock in. It is one of the easiest positions for a novice to be fucked in: The penetration of the cock up his asshole is not as deep as in several

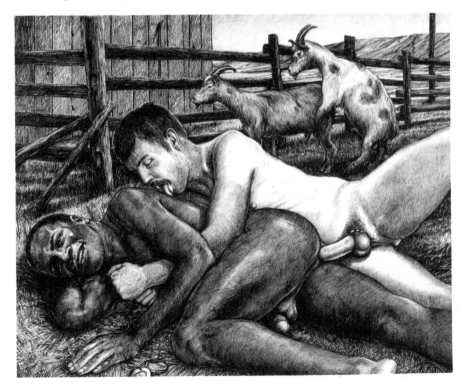

others (see *Face-to-Face; Sitting on It*); he is not as immobile as when he is lying flat on his stomach. Nor is his own cock inaccessible. In fact, the man doing the fucking can easily wrap his arms around his partner and masturbate and fondle him.

SIT ON MY FACE

his polite imperative, offering comfort and pleasure, is hard to resist. Gay men spend a lot of time on their buns at the gym, and buying just the right pants to show them off. Gay men's tongues have also learned to explore these exotic regions. From the grasslands of armpits, down to the subtropical balls—this is as far a journey as some tongues used to take. But nowadays the adventurous tongue's trip around the world would be incomplete without a visit to that tropical rain forest of the human body—that land of perpetual moisture, tangled vegetation, and exotic smells: the asshole and environs.

As the eminent English poet W. H. Auden says:

I've often thought that I would like
To be the saddle on a bike.

Whether you are the sitter or the seat, it's a delicate and intimate maneuver. Get into position gradually, taking into account each other's weight, size, and flexibility, or else the man on the bottom will find his eyes, nose and mouth pressed, squeezed, and sealed shut. If you just plop down, the partner beneath you will writhe hysterically, fearing imminent asphyxiation, while your ass will feel as if it is being attacked by gnawing rodents escaping a trap. For some men, the thrill of the experience lies in submission to the weight and smell and oxygen-blocking properties of their partner's body. For others, the turn-on is inflicting humiliation as their bottom becomes literally their ass-kisser.

But for many, there is something very tender and intimate and delicate about the pleasure of this trip. Before he actually sits on your face, try this. Put him on his back with his legs over his head. Make sure your face is wet with saliva. Close your eyes and mouth, and rub your face in one long motion from the small of his back, up his crack, all the way across his rectum and up over his balls. With a little practice you will be able to end up with your head upside down on his belly and your mouth on his dick.

Have him straddle your chest on his knees, facing your feet, while he lowers his butt over your face. In this position you can keep one hand on his belly and cock, and one hand on his ass to steady his weight, while he can reach your cock with his hands and his mouth. You'll have tantalizing glimpses up his tensed, straining back as your tongue and lips and teeth dart around. If he moves up a bit and sits on your forehead he can rub his buns hard on your brow while you lick his balls. Or, if you want a better view, guide him, taking his open hand and slapping yourself with it until he gets the picture.

Most men who like a little ass-slapping integrate it into the full menu of sex. For other men, spanking is the full meal. The spanking scene often (but not always) occurs within a "Daddy" fantasy of punishing or rewarding a boy (see *Daddy-Son Fantasies*). Another popular spanking fantasy is the frat-house scenario. In this fantasy the sex partners act out scenes where one is the freshman, pledging the fraternity, who is spanked, paddled, and sometimes forced into sexually servicing the frat-house senior, all as part of the accepted hazing ritual. There are a variety of porno videos, as well as special magazines and newsletters, devoted to spanking.

STAND AND DELIVER

Fucking someone while you are both standing, his back to you, may be required when trying to make it in a confined vertical space. At home it adds to the excitement if you're surrounded by mirrors so you can see your interlocked bodies from every angle. It also helps if the man getting fucked leans forward and braces his weight against the wall (or mirror) with his hands. That way he's firmly anchored and can push back. If there is a difference in size between the fucker and fuckee, standing on something steady will balance it out.

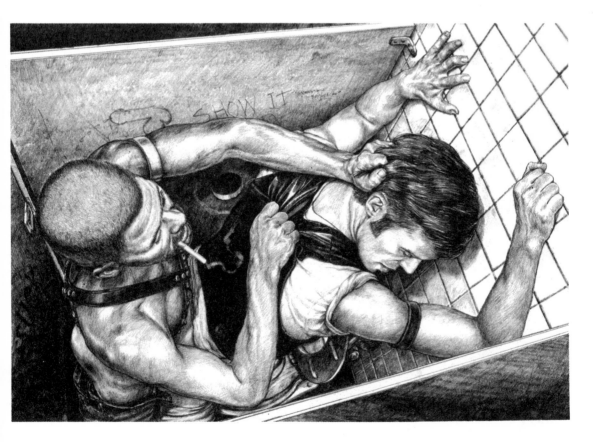

While this position doesn't at first seem to offer the intimacy of other positions, it can still be quite a turn-on if the man in back, doing the fucking, nibbles, kisses, and bites at the back and sides of his partner's neck. He can also caress his partner's chest and play with his nipples. Some guys really love receiving this kind of attention: They can get fucked and simultaneously jerk themselves off, while all the while being securely held and fondled by their partner.

A fun variation is to lift your partner into the air from behind, while fucking him. You can also do this if you're facing, his arms wrapped around your neck and his legs around your waist. Anyone who has experienced an orgasm in midair while being fucked will confirm that it is a unique pleasure. Sometimes called air express, this is even better in a three-way if you are being sucked off, say, while being fucked from behind (see *Three-ways*). And this is yet another advantage of the stand-and-deliver position: In sex scenes involving more than two people, it's ideal—not only as outlined above, but, for example, getting fucked while you're sucking off someone else, while you yourself are being sucked off by someone kneeling in front of you. The permutations are only limited by imagination and the space.

SUICIDE

Some gay men who are either seropositive or showing symptoms of HIV Disease think about suicide. At first, it's only a vague thought, but later, when serious illnesses invade the body, they wonder at what point life becomes more painful than death. Some of us are more upset by our increased dependence upon lovers, friends, or family than by the actual illnesses. The prouder the man, the more uncomfortable it may be for him to feel like a burden. Such men may consider destroying themselves in order to preserve their sense of personal dignity. It's as if they are saying, "I'm the one who's going to make the important decisions about my life, not this illness or doctors." This decision to take control makes them psychologically stronger.

Self-destruction can occur when a person feels helpless, hopeless, loveless—thoroughly defeated by life. Talking about these feelings with a trusted friend or lover restores emotional attachments. *If you discuss the problem with someone close, suicide becomes both less terrifying and less likely, though it remains an option.* Sometimes, people feel timid and incompetent when a friend or lover talks about suicide. The best advice is: Talk openly with your friend about his fantasies of self-destruction, and express your own feelings about it. Don't be afraid that you'll say the wrong thing or that you'll push him over the edge. You won't. Only he can decide for himself. Someone close to the PWA (person with AIDS) should contact a local AIDS service organization, or, if needed, a therapist can be consulted who can treat the depression.

Gay teenagers are also prone to suicide. The Centers for Disease Control has studied adolescent suicide and come up with a truly gut-wrenching statistic: Fully one third of all teenagers who kill themselves are gay.

It's not difficult to understand the prevalence of gay teen suicide. Being gay at this age can be traumatic in our society (see *Teenagers*). High-school counselors are generally as homophobic as the general population. Their main aim is getting the teen to conform, i.e., to be less openly gay.

The CDC notes three special danger signs that a teenager may kill himself. First, if he is gay-identified from preadolescence, he faces bigotry, ostracism, and violence early in his life. Second, effeminacy adds an additional burden of stress because of teasing by peers and adults. Third, if the boy gets crushes on other boys, he will encounter constant rejection. Most gay teens run into so much bigotry that it only deepens their sense of alienation. Even when a gay teen does find a lover, the two may feel so alone and harassed that they form a suicide pact.

If you are a gay teen who is considering suicide, call your local lesbian/gay switchboard (look it up in the telephone book). The people on the switchboard or from local groups like the Samaritans (212-673-3000) are nonjudgmental, anonymous volunteers. They will talk to you and help you.

TEAROOMS AND BACK ROOMS

"Tearoom" is the slang term used by gays for any public toilet where men engage in sex. Every town seems to have at least one "notorious" tearoom—at the bus station, at a rest stop on the highway, in the public library, at a subway stop, in the student union. Gays who have traveled in Eastern Europe have reported that the safest and most active tearooms were formerly found very close to Communist or police headquarters.

Pay toilets are preferred, since the rattle of the coin in the outside door slot serves as a warning to the men already inside the toilet and gives them time to pull up their pants before someone (especially a policeman) walks in.

The etiquette of tearoom sex is elaborate. Two men stand side by side at a urinal. Each gets a hard-on. If no one else is around, they reach for each other. If other people are present and are just standing around, they are presumably gay and sympathetic.

Cruising from one toilet stall to another has its own rituals. In some cases, small holes have been pierced through the partitions (sometimes through a slab of marble. When? Using what tools?). One man looks through the hole and sees another playing with himself. One may stand to give a better view of his erect cock. Then the process is reversed. In some tearooms the hole is large enough to stick a cock through; such "glory holes" are used for giving and receiving blow jobs. If there are no holes in the partition the men may begin a "tap dance." Jack taps with his shoe. Bill taps back. Jack inches his shoe toward Bill's; then Bill's shoe moves in Jack's direction. Eventually shoes touch. Bill reaches under the partition, and Jack squats so Bill can grab his cock. Then Jack reaches under and feels Bill up. Finally Jack shoves as far as possible under the partition and Bill sucks him off, or vice versa. Or one man passes the other a note scribbled on toilet paper: "Do you have a place? Do you have time? What do you look like? Are you hairy? Hung? What are you into? The questionnaires can rival the U.S. Army's for details requested.

Tearooms can be very dangerous. Policemen, either in uniform or in plain clothes, keep tabs on them and sometimes videotape or observe the activities from concealed vantage points. The police in some towns entrap gays by initiating sex, then flashing a badge just as the man is about to go down on the officer (or just after he's finished sucking the cop off).

Most municipalities have laws against public sex, so you're never safe in a tearoom, and you're especially vulnerable if you're inexperienced and not tuned in to danger signals. One signal: You start fooling around with a guy whose heart is pounding and who can't get an erection; he might be anxious, or he may be about to rob you. Often, hoodlums and petty thugs corner a gay man after soliciting him in a tearoom, rob him, and beat him up. If you have any doubt at all, move away, zip up, and get out.

Because of their ubiquity on the American scene, tearooms have been the subject of sociological study, some of which is quite enlightening. (Read *Tearoom Trade* by Laud Humphreys.) Many of the habitués of tearooms turn out to be "straight"—i.e., married or closeted gay men who, to hide their homosexuality, will not be seen in a public gay bar, club, or restaurant. The age range, depending on the specific tearoom, can be anywhere from the teens to the seventies.

The sexual reciprocation in tearooms is as often on a chain basis as it is one-to-one. That is to say, Mark sucks off Bill, who leaves. Terry, who was perhaps watching that encounter, then sucks off Mark, who leaves, and so on. Three-ways and orgies are also not uncommon in tearooms (see *Orgies; Three-ways*).

The most active tearooms—after work, during lunch—usually develop "monitors," men who do nothing sexually but watch other men have sex. They stand at the entry and monitor those approaching; they warn of a policeman, teen thugs, or anyone suspicious. Before the toilets were closed, elaborately detailed maps of the New York City subway system were prepared by tearoom mavens, complete with comments on the best times to visit and the kinds of people to be found there. Some even specifically named men who might be met at any one of the hundreds of station johns in the system.

Back rooms are dark places in gay bars or clubs where men have sex. Back rooms were the liberated gay male's answer to tearooms in the late sixties through the eighties, but because of health reasons they are far less common today. These rooms are so dark you can scarcely see whom you're fucking or sucking. If you meet someone terrific in a back room, you can always whisper an invitation to come home, though you may be in for a surprise (pleasant or otherwise) when you see him in the light.

Back rooms are much less hazardous than tearooms. There's virtually no chance that the police will bust you or that a mugger will beat you up. But pickpockets routinely lift wallets in the obscurity of back rooms, and the places can be breeding grounds for disease. Be sure to leave your money, identification, and credit cards at home, or hide them in the bottom of your shoe. Unfortunately, like sex clubs, they are fast becoming unsafe environments (see *Sex Clubs*).

TEENAGERS

Some boys know they're gay from a very early age. For others, their sexual interests only become apparent with the onset of puberty. In coming out, both these groups of young people run up against significant obstacles, not the least of which is avoiding the condemnation of parents and other adults (see *Coming Out; Parents*).

Some youngsters look for sex with boys their own age. The first Kinsey Report, which shocked the nation in 1948, found that about one-third of the researchers' sample of men had had a homosexual experience to orgasm. Perhaps much of this sex consisted of two or more boys jacking off together, since "getting your rocks off" has always been acceptable male behavior.

Some teenagers also fall in love with an age-mate. Here one finds deep emotional attachments. These love affairs between gay boys usually don't last very long because they are vulnerable to exposure and punishment. Subject to alternating high and low moods, adolescents often end up severely depressed. Occasionally one hears about adolescents who commit double suicide, and one wonders whether they were lovers who saw no other choice in a prejudiced world that forbids their love (see *Suicide*).

If you are a teenager looking for sex or romance with other teens, we have good news—and we have bad news. The good news is that many high schools and colleges now have gay/lesbian clubs. There's even the Harvey Milk School, an accredited high school in New York City, for gay kids. Big cities have gay youth groups (get their phone number through your gay hot line or look them up in the *Gayellow Pages*). At your age, it is crucial to learn that you're not alone. You'll meet new friends and learn about their lives, hopes, and fears, which may turn out to be exactly like your own. Other gay teens will also provide you with needed support when everyone else is putting you down for being who you are.

Sometimes you can't find a friend or sympathetic ear. A book may become your friend and teacher. Many excellent books (novels such as

Sandra Scoppetone's *Trying Hard to Hear You* and true stories like Aaron Fricke's *Reflections of a Rock Lobster*) have been written about and for gay teenagers. If these aren't in your local library or bookstore, try to locate them through gay mail-order catalogues, although if you order them, be certain that your mail is secure from prying eyes.

And now the bad news. Coming out during the AIDS crisis is very difficult. It means that you are required to practice safe sex with all your sexual partners. We know that this is a hard burden for teenagers to accept. But practicing safe sex is an indication of both your respect for yourself and your respect for others. No gay person should put either his own life or another person's life in jeopardy (see *Condoms; Dangerous Sex; Lubricants; Safe Sex; Saying No*).

There are some teenagers who prefer sex with adults. They do so for a number of reasons. Instead of bumbling around with friends their own age, they want a man who is sexually experienced and will patiently teach them. Looking for an appropriate role model is another reason. A few others, particularly those from poor or dysfunctional families, have sex with adults for money. Finally, there are adolescents who are looking for an affectionate gay man as a replacement for an unloving (often a cruel) father.

If you are a teenager interested in adults, please understand that while some of them may be attracted to you, few will actually have sex with you. Outside of special circumstances, most men (gay or straight) are wary of a boy's sexual interest. Society has historically been ruthless toward men it considers child molesters. If you are below the age of consent and looking for sex, be aware that your adult sex partner, if caught, could end up in prison for a very long time.

Many adults angrily reject the possibility that adolescents can and do regularly consent to sex with adults. They insist that any sexual contact between a teenager and an adult is exploitative—regardless of what the youngster's desires are. They believe this even in the face of evidence of intergenerational sex that led to long-lasting love. One of the authors met a couple who had been lovers for fifty years; they first met at the unusual ages of eleven and twenty-one. How many intergenerational love affairs exist today is unknown.

Most teenagers worry more about coming out to their families than about sex (see *Parents*). Parents are more sympathetic toward their gay kids these days than ever before. Many of these enlightened parents will also welcome a lover into their home during holidays. Be advised, however, that your parents are going to be very worried about HIV Disease and your health. If you come out to them, be prepared to talk about safe sex, and to reassure them that you intend to remain healthy (see *HIV Disease; Sexually Transmitted Diseases*). Unfortunately, some parents do reject their gay sons. Gay teenage runaways exist in large numbers because their parents abused them, sexually molested them, or kicked them out. These teenagers usually report that being kicked out was the least difficult part, because

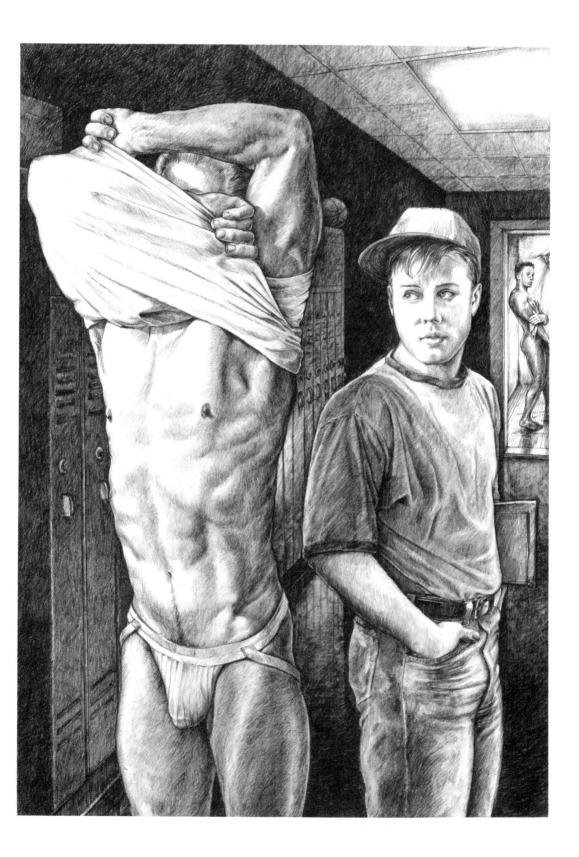

living at home had become such a horror show. But it's very difficult being a runaway. There are psychopathic adults who exploit runaways by introducing them to drugs and prostitution. Even when runaway teenagers manage to band together, it's very hard to survive without a home and money. Illness and despair can destroy the tightest of friendships.

The biggest cities, where runaways tend to gravitate, also have the most programs to help runaway teens. They're not perfect, and are always underfunded, but the workers there genuinely care for kids. If they didn't, they'd be working elsewhere. Try Covenant House (800-999-9999) in New York City, or your local lesbian/gay switchboard.

TENDERNESS

There are some men who just want sex, but most of us want more—we want tenderness. There are times when our sexual desires feel like nothing more than an itch that needs to be scratched, and no tenderness is involved. When tenderness *is* involved, sex is not an isolated event but the continuation of a long, lively dialogue.

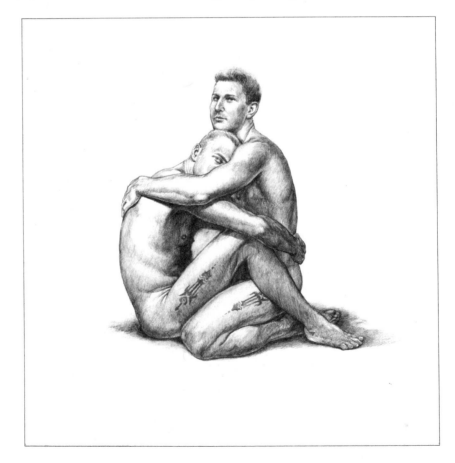

Tenderness is based on communication. If you are attentive and responsive to your partner's sexual needs, even when he needs to be handled roughly, then you are tender. Although tenderness can be gentle, it need not be. Whether the touch is soft or rough, tenderness is expressed when you evaluate the needs of your partner and meet them—and when you allow him to meet yours.

If you are cold and indifferent to your partner, or if you establish a narrow, mechanical sexual program for your encounters with him, one that disregards his moods and taste for variety, then you are not being tender. And if you refuse to express your own sexual needs and insist on only servicing his, then you are also guilty of a lack of tenderness (see *Pleasure Trap*).

Tenderness requires that you understand the rhythm of sexual passion —that you indulge in foreplay, that you pick up signals, that you accommodate yourself to your partner's predilections, and that after sex you assure him of your affection. Newcomers to sex can learn the various positions easily enough; what requires patience is the acquisition of tenderness. It comes only with experience.

THREE-WAYS

A three-way adds spice to home cooking by throwing in a new flavor. It can also be satisfying when the participants have just met. The best three-ways occur when all members are sexually versatile.

A man in the proper mood can get his face and his ass fucked simultaneously. Or he can kneel, and suck both his buddies simultaneously while they stand and kiss. One man can fuck a second lying on his back, and while fucking he can suck a third who's standing. Or the two doing the fucking can simultaneously suck off the third, who at the same time may be opposite them in bed, kissing, caressing, or even sucking the genitalia of one or both of them.

Some men are able to get fucked by two cocks at once. One man may like to watch his lover fucking someone else, especially if he can't get fucked by his lover himself or finds getting fucked more exciting an idea than a reality. Another may like to fuck and get fucked simultaneously, once he's gotten the pelvic motions coordinated.

Three-ways aren't always problem-free. It's not unusual for one participant to become jealous or feel left out. Some lovers think a three-way would be nifty, but when it comes to execution one of them turns possessive and brooding. If three strangers are involved, two may hit it off so well they want to be alone, and the third feels he's just being used. If three-ways are the only sex lovers do anymore, they could fall into a pat routine, mechanical in its action (pairs have been known to call out numbers, like gridiron quarterbacks, signifying, say, time for all to suck).

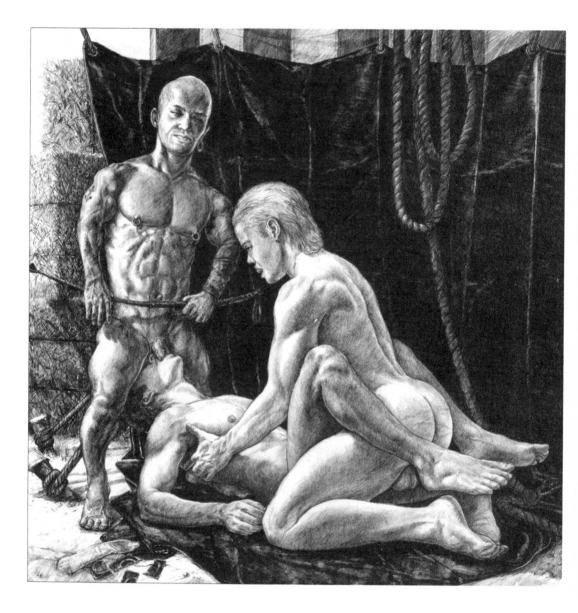

If all goes well, however, a three-way can be exhilarating and surprisingly intimate. After three men have explored every possible sensual aspect and sexual potentiality of one another's bodies in every conceivable combination, they often lie around and talk for hours, suffused with a warm glow. At times three-ways seem so natural one wonders why lovers don't come in threes more often.

The answer is that once love and romance have been added into the pot, the simple three-way becomes the far more complex triangle. While love triangles are responsible for much of the world's great literature (not to mention most daily gossip), triangles require the utmost of intelligence, affection, common sense, a selflessness to pull off. Even then, few triangles last over a period of time without major adjustments in all three lovers' minds and lives.

T O P

Being known as a top (see *Bottom*) can be helpful in meeting potential sex partners. People not interested in being bottoms automatically eliminate themselves, while those interested let it be known. It's also useful when placing ads (see *Sex Ads*). Being a top does not mean that you're more desirable than a bottom. It also doesn't mean that you must rigidly remain in that role or that you can't get fucked if you like. Assuming you practice safe sex, feel free to alternate top and bottom according to the situation or your partner.

There are differences, though, between tops and bottoms. The top, for example, would seem to be the protector, the controller, the one who does the bulk of the leading and guiding, the one who takes on the responsibilities.

Ironically, before the Stonewall riots, when gays were far more closeted than today, roles like top and bottom were more rigid because gay men felt required to assume invariable roles. In a sense, it was a mirror of heterosexual role playing, the bottom assuming a femalelike persona, while the top was the man (see *Gay Liberation*). Terms like "butch" and "femme" were common appellations for American gay men describing themselves up to the sixties. One still hears these terms used by some gay men and lesbians.

Memoirs and interviews with gays who flourished in earlier decades make those distinctions clear. As a rule, femmes lived more or less openly gay lives. They dressed in "womanish" slacks and fluffy mohair sweaters; their hair was cut in gender-ambiguous styles. They often wore makeup. They paid dearly for this freedom: They were discriminated against severely, even by other gays (see *Effeminacy*). They worked in gay occupations such as hairdressing, theatrical costuming, and interior decoration, or in low-paying jobs inside the tiny gay ghettos of New York and San Francisco, as stage dancers, waiters, and shop clerks.

The butch gay could be in any profession, from sanitation man to company CEO, since he was passing for straight. He never allowed himself a "feminine" action, except when very disinhibited by liquor or drugs, and only in the most secure gay company. Unlike the femme, he had the freedom to live and work wherever he chose.

The American public of the first half of this century only recognized femmes as gay, never butches. But femmes also used this instant recognition. They could have "straight" male admirers and boyfriends—especially if they were themselves rich, powerful, or beautiful or if they were in glamour fields like cinema, music, and show business.

The gay men who came out around the time of the Stonewall riots wanted to lock butch and femme role-playing into the closet of history forever. The gay liberationists' point was that all gays, no matter what their specific sexual behavior, were men. As a result of the surprising success of the gay movement, butch gays became free to try new roles, while effeminate gays found themselves politically passé. Yet it's interesting to note that political correctness hasn't changed the fact that gay men have sexual preferences. The terms "top" and "bottom" no longer convey a heterosexual dichotomy of husband and wife, as "butch" and "femme" did. Even so, while some men easily move from one to the other, most gay men have a preference for one over the other. It's perfectly normal to be solidly top or bottom.

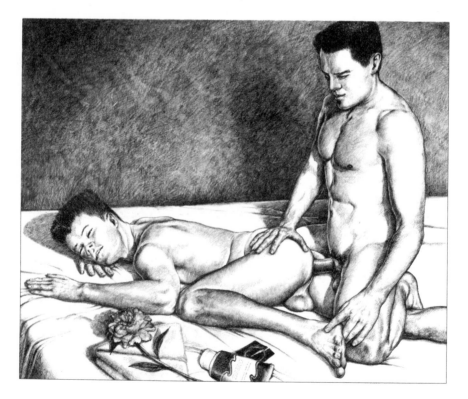

TOUCHING AND HOLDING

Of all the means of communication, touch is by far the most sensitive. Through touch the child learns either to trust or to mistrust other people around him, and consequently touch and trust become intimately related.

Some of us become elegant in speech, charmers who use our verbal facilities to hide our feelings as often as to express them. Other men, less competent verbally, fine-tune their hands and know how to please other men sexually. Lucky for us to find a lover skilled at both.

The problem with touch is that it often conveys the truth about one's feelings, rather than the lie one is telling. In other words, people "read" communication by touch as more truthful than that by speech. They're usually right.

There are a number of components of touch as a communicator of our feelings. Softness conveys closeness, but hardness expresses anger or resentment. The speed of our touch is another obvious indicator. A quick cuddle or massage is tantamount to saying "Let's get this over with because I'd rather do something else." How many fingers one uses while touching is also important. We all know that the tips of our fingers are the most sensitive areas, and using them—all of them—expresses our desire to remain in contact with our partner.

There are times when we use touch like a lie-detector test. The hand may be touching and caressing us, but we notice our lover's arm fully extended and the rest of his body far away. Physical distance during touch may express conflicts in the people's feelings toward each other. Commonly, while a man's words are affectionate, his touching expresses his ambivalence about the relationship.

Touch becomes more varied when our lover is willing to touch with his tongue and mouth, and for us to do the same to him. Part of the fun of being lovers is to explore with hand, tongue, and mouth every inch of your partner's skin, and to find the special spots that encourage him to squirm with pleasure.

Occasionally we find a lover who pleases us completely. He's usually a man in whom one finds a congruence of words and touch. Whether for just a night or for a lifetime, we feel safe in his arms. While we can't all meet that standard, we can learn to become better at touch, and at communicating in general.

Here's a good touching exercise to do with a partner.

You'll need a long stretch of uninterrupted time, so turn on your answering machine. Take showers, and clear your minds of work or other outside activities. Let's say you're going to pleasure your partner first. He should get naked and lie on his back. You have a choice of starting at his head and working down to his toes, or the other way around. Your object is to gently caress every square inch of his skin. If you're starting at his feet, caress every toe, the soles of his feet, the sides, and work your way up the foot slowly. Sometimes you'll use just a few fingers, sometimes a whole hand, and when appropriate, both hands. Use your imagination. Play with his hair, and lightly pinch his skin if you wish. Use your tongue and mouth whenever and wherever you want. Except—you are not to give him a blow job. No orgasms! Otherwise you'd interrupt the exercise midway. Naturally he'll have a hard-on. Let it be. Feel free to stop and play at any interesting spot, say his belly button or the hair just below it, his nipples or earlobes. Touch them, lick them, suck them—and at some point touch and lick at the same time.

When you've finished one side of his body, turn him over and slowly and gently do the other side. Pay particular attention to his butt. Spread the cheeks and rub your nose around the crack. Wet all the hair by drenching the area with saliva, but don't do any rimming. If the tropical forest around his butt hole isn't your cup of tea, then skip it (see *Rimming*).

If you're the one being touched, your only responsibility is to lie there and enjoy it. Ironically, that's a problem for lots of men, because we're so used to being in control that passivity makes us anxious. If one kind of touch is uncomfortable, tell him so (see *Massage*).

The whole exercise could take an hour or more. When it's finished, lie together in bed, touching each other gently. One or the other may feel the need to be held. Some couples like to have sex afterward; others avoid it. Do as the two of you wish. The next time you do this touching exercise, switch roles.

People who are HIV-positive or who have HIV Disease also need to be touched. Their need is even greater than it is for the rest of us, because they fear being abandoned by friends and family. The touching exercise described above can and should be done with them because there are no physical dangers to it. Some gay men fear physical closeness to a friend with HIV Disease, for a variety of reasons. The first is obviously fear of contamination. It's a primitive fear of being harmed, even though the well person knows that the virus isn't transmitted casually. Some eschew contact because they're afraid of finding a friend dependent upon them. There are also those men who simply feel incompetent to express their warmth and compassion for a friend. Yet those who touch, hug, and cuddle with their ill friends invariably leave feeling enriched by the experience, while the ill friends become energized, feeling cared for by a world that is slowly slipping from their grasp.

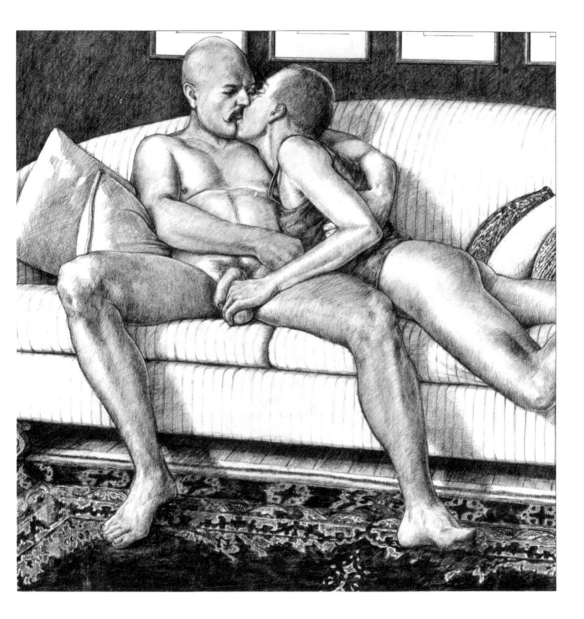

TRADE

Men who are (or pretend to be) straight will sometimes allow a gay man to suck them off. These men are called *trade*. The word may be confusing when first heard, since it suggests reciprocity, which is not generally the case. Sometimes there is an exchange, since hustlers are paid for the use of their bodies.

In gay slang, "trade" crops up in many contexts. "Just let me do you for trade," one gay might say, half-humorously, to another who has rejected him. Translation: "You don't have to do anything except lie back and let me blow you."

Someone straight and potentially dangerous is called rough trade. Hustlers are known as commercial trade. Both terms naturally connote danger. Two constants emerge: He who is "trade" plays the straight role, and the sex is geared to his climax, not to mutual orgasm.

Why does the concept of trade continue to persist long after Stonewall and gay liberation? Is it that the gay man who habitually gives the blow jobs is someone who hates his own homosexuality and prefers to identify with a "real man"? Or is the man who's trade himself afraid of losing his masculine image and becoming a "faggot," and his pose a defense?

Possibly. Perhaps for the gay man, self-abasement before an ostensibly heterosexual man may have come to seem deeply erotic, or perhaps the gay man is sexually conditioned to humiliation. Hostility intermingled with sexual excitement may motivate both parties: The trade feels contempt for the faggot servicing him and the faggot feels contempt for the straight man whose heterosexuality is so easily bypassed. More often these days, being trade is a mask for the man's internalized homophobia, and he pretends to do it for money, not because he likes it (see *Homophobia*). Hence the old adage "Today's trade is tomorrow's competition."

Yet another widespread usage of "trade" relates to a teenager or young man who is experimenting with his homosexuality or bisexuality, and who wishes to experience as much as possible with little change to his self-image. Being trade, he can associate with gays, learn about gay life, and discover what will be required of him socially as well as sexually should he come out.

TRANSVESTITES AND TRANSSEXUALS

Cross-dressing is not a new phenomenon. It's been around for ages. Joan of Arc, for example, was the most prominent transvestite of the fifteenth century. She was tried for dressing like a man (a capital crime in her day) and was burned at the stake.

France had many transvestites, some of them members of the royal family. "Monsieur," the brother of King Louis XIV, was probably the most famous. A superb general, he fought in full drag under his armor and complained that the smoke of battle messed up his makeup. The eighteenth-century Chevalier d'Eon de Beaumont (during the reign of Louis XV) was denounced as a hermaphrodite by a political enemy. Members of the court were so confused about his real sex that they laid bets and planned to kidnap him to settle the question, but he evaded them. Confessing to the king that he was a woman, he was ordered to wear women's clothes for the rest of his life. He then started giving fencing lessons while dressed as a woman. When he died in 1810 he was found to be a perfectly formed man.

Though transvestites and transsexuals have often banded together for political purposes, they are quite distinct. *Transvestites* are men who dress up as women. The majority of all transvestites are heterosexuals with no sexual interest in other men. The term was coined in this century by the famous German sex researcher Magnus Hirschfeld. (Read *Transvestism: The Erotic Drive to Cross-dress* by Magnus Hirschfeld.)

Homosexual transvestites are called drag queens, either with respect or, by some, with contempt. They, in turn, often call other gay men butch queens. More recently the term "transgender" has been used. Gay transvestites are poorly understood and are mistreated by most of the male population; they must endure not only the jeers of straights but also the put-downs of some other gays. In certain bars, transvestites are called upon to host a party, emcee a show, or lip-synch a song by Garland or Streisand. Being gregarious, they're often the social glue in the place. They are prominent participants in gay liberation parades.

Gay transvestites cross-dress for many different reasons. Some dress as men in public and wear drag only at home or during private parties. Others lead a double life, wearing male costume on the job and female attire at all other times. There are also transvestites who are so accomplished in their dress and manner that they live publicly as women. Some are so convincing that they work in what are thought of as specifically women's trades. For instance La Putassa was a famous drag fashion model of the eighties, and one Rio de Janeiro beauty named Roberto/Roberta was even Miss Brazil in the Miss Universe contest.

For some the great drag event is an annual ball. Many transvestites spend an entire year and a small fortune designing and assembling their gowns for these occasions. The costumes can be miracles of invention: One year the winner of a New Orleans Mardi Gras contest was carried to the judges' stand in a gilded cage, which at the climactic moment sprang open, releasing hundreds of birds—and the drag artist, in a fantasy of feathers. An excellent, prize-winning film about drags and drag balls, *Paris Is Burning*, shows this life, especially among African-American and Latino drags, with great style, verve, humor, and understanding. Their drag balls are highly creative and feature men's business suits as costumes as often as cross-dressing. The balls are produced by "houses," which are organized like families whose members represent the house when competing in the balls. Not surprisingly, each family has a mother and father, who lead and advise other family members.

Transvestism bears little relationship to sexual behavior. Gay transvestites can be surprisingly aggressive in sex, or versatile in fucking or being fucked. Some live as wives, both socially and sexually, with "butch" husbands. While some transvestites are conventionally moral, others are prostitutes. Although a few gay transvestites long to have a sex change, most are happy about having it both ways.

Drag queens, particularly those who come from a working-class background, can be very tough. They've had to survive the prejudice against them. It was drag queens and street hustlers who began the riots at the Stonewall (see *Gay Liberation*). Afterward the TVs (as they sometimes refer to themselves) formed STAR (Street Transvestite Action Revolutionaries), which was one of the gutsiest groups in gay political demonstrations. Drags are justifiably resentful that they are not given credit for their contributions and have been pushed aside by straighter-looking gay men, many of whom consider drags an embarrassment to the gay struggle.

On the other hand, *transsexuals* have an unshakable conviction (dating from childhood) that fate played some dreadful prank on them by bringing them into the world as men. They sometimes feel like feminine dryads trapped within masculine bark; they long to be released. Several medical centers, both in the United States and abroad, have helped these men to make the transition from male to female. Oddly, the number of medical institutions performing these operations has declined in the last decade.

The first recorded sex reassignment we know of was performed in 1882 on Sophia Hedwig, who changed her name to Herman Karl. With medical help she grew a beard, and surgeons tried to fashion her a set of testicles, a scrotum, and a penis. We don't know whether the surgery was successful or how her later life went. The term "transsexual" first appears in the scientific literature in 1949, coined by Cauldwell in *Sexology* magazine. Then Dr. Harry Benjamin became the most prominent authority on and the person most associated with the phenomenon.

Because it is so socially, emotionally, and physically complex, and because it is irreversible, the complete process of sex reassignment can often take years. First, the client is given an extensive psychological examination. He will probably begin counseling or psychotherapy, to deal with the emotional aspects of reassignment from male to female. His beard is removed by electrolysis, and he starts receiving female hormones (which he must continue to take forever). The hormones cause the breasts to swell, the hair to acquire a new luster, the body to become softer and more curvaceous, and the hips to enlarge. Hormone treatment generally continues for a period of one or two years. During this time, the client and his therapist evaluate the progress made in the transition from male to female. Some transsexuals decide to go no further than hormone treatment. Most request the final stage of treatment: surgical reassignment. Through an extensive set of operations, the scrotum is removed, as is most of the penis. Portions of the latter—the sensitive glans and the urethra—are retained to form the new clitoris and top inner wall of the new vagina. Other procedures include cosmetic facial surgery—such as shaving down the Adam's apple—intended to soften and demasculinize the appearance. If all goes well, the sexually reassigned man looks like and responds sexually as a woman. There are, in fact, quite a few transsexuals whose husbands remain unaware that their wives are genetically male. The secret is sometimes disclosed when the question of having children arises. Transsexuals are incapable of bearing children.

The entire reassignment procedure, from the initial consultation to the final operation, is expensive both financially and psychologically. Medical insurance will not pay for most of the treatments, and considerable absences from work can be expected. The psychological problems include reestablishing relationships with family members and friends and accepting the emotional difficulties that reassignment brings. (Read *The Uninvited Dilemma: The Question of Gender* by Kim Stuart.)

Many gay men do not accept transsexualism as a bona fide phenomenon. They believe, wrongly, that a transsexual is a man who suffers from so extreme a form of internalized homophobia that he's willing to sacrifice his genitalia. Transsexuals therefore become a sexual minority who are rejected even by other sexual minorities. Still, even though often dismissed by both gay and straight people, many of them complete reassignment and live productive lives.

TRICKING

There are periods in a gay man's life when he feels like having a lot of sex with many different guys. Generally, although not always, this period comes right after a young man has accepted his homosexuality, or when he has broken out of a difficult and lingering relationship. It can happen when you leave home for college, leave college for work, move to a new town, take a new job, come into money, or lose a parent who never approved of your gay life. It could even happen if you're fired from your job or if you lose an important social position. You find yourself with time on your hands; you feel frustrated or, more often, feel an extra surge of libido.

The word "tricking" comes from prostitutes' slang, and signifies having sex with a paying client, known as the trick or john. Making such a date is called turning a trick. In gay life we've shortened it to "tricking."

Gays adopted the term possibly because they associated with prostitutes. Since the sexual revolution of the sixties and seventies, a new term

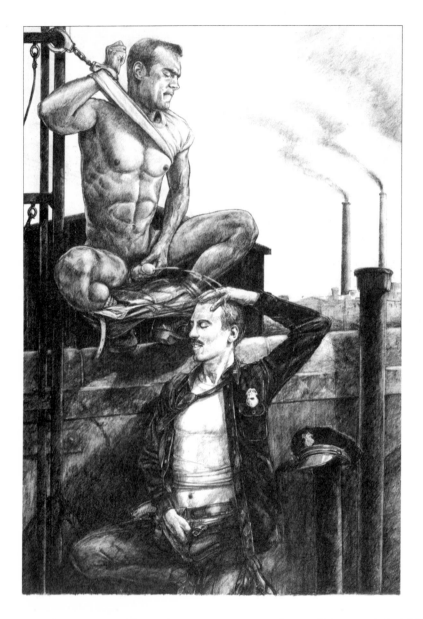

has come into usage without the accompanying stigma of the word ''trick''
—''one-night stand''; it's used by gays and straights alike.

''One-night stand'' signifies that two people who've just met plan to
spend a limited time together during which they'll have sex. If this occurs
at one of the two partners' homes, the encounter is not expected to last
beyond the next morning. As likely, one partner will leave after sex, perhaps
after having exchanged phone numbers and promises to call. Implicit in the
idea of the one-night stand is that if the pair like each other enough, they'll
spend a second night together, a third, perhaps more.

A great deal has been written about how shallow and vapid one-night stands are, how geared to the "consumer society"—just "fast-food sex." All of these criticisms seem apt.

On the other hand, if people are not looking for commitment, and they'd like to have sex with many people, and they are healthy, prudent, and safe, *why not* trick around? Who's being hurt?

Probably no one. The person tricking gets to spend time with a variety of people and to learn how to handle himself in a variety of situations. Perhaps he wants to taste many physical types from chubby to Adonis, from effeminate queen to biker leatherman, from milk-skinned blond to ebony-skinned African-American (see *Types*). What better way than tricking to carry on your own Study of Man? Or he might want to experiment with different sexual roles (see *Bottom; Role-playing; Sadomasochism*).

And tricks can turn into lovers, friends, business associates, doctors, lawyers, customers. Many older gays swear that the years they were tricking around formed a social network for the rest of their lives, and taught them how to handle themselves socially.

That's the good part. On the other hand, you can hurt yourself tricking around if: 1) You can't stop yourself; 2) you've met someone you like a lot but you won't see him a second or third time because there might be someone even better out there; or 3) you've begun a relationship with someone, but as soon as difficulties arise, you quickly bow out, telling yourself, "I don't need this hassle, I can have sex whenever I want."

Once tricking becomes obsessive behavior out of which you gain less and less pleasure, *then* it's hurting you.

Until then, be safe, be careful, and enjoy yourself.

(See *Cruising; Promiscuity; Safe Sex; Seduction*.)

TYPES

We often forget that most people have physical types that they definitely prefer. The African-American guy you're so hot for may have turned you down because you're white; study him a few nights and you'll probably notice he leaves only with other blacks. The cowboy who turned you down probably did so because you're dark and tall; observe, and you will doubtless see he's always got a small blond in tow. The cultivated balletomane with whom you discussed Baryshnikov and Jerry Robbins's latest with such pleasure more than likely didn't go home with you because he's only turned on by monosyllabic morons.

Spare yourself grief: Recognize that you are not the universal solvent, no matter how attractive you may be. No one is. Even your assets may work against you: Your perfect features and bulging biceps may intimidate men who feel more comfortable with ordinary looks. Conversely, what you may label your flaws may constitute your chief appeal to others: Your beard grew in bicolored, black and ginger, which you consider a tragedy, but it may be irresistible to some men, especially to those who like "bears" (see *New Macho Images*).

There's another dimension to the subject of types: How do you avoid being type*cast*? Sexual proclivities seldom conform to appearance. A small, cuddly young man may like to dominate others in bed. A muscular, over-sized guy may tire of having his smaller, slimmer tricks demand that he ravish them. A slender Asian may not want to always play the shy geisha; a man in his sixties may not like to play Daddy every night. If you find yourself trapped by others' stereotypes of you, the best move you can make is to state or demonstrate your desires explicitly. On the other hand, you've got to be willing to stop dressing and behaving in a way that arouses stereotypical—and, in your case, false—expectations. If you look like a cute kid, and dress the part, you succeed in getting lots of attention. If you depart from this look you may be less popular. No matter. What's the use of awakening desire in others, if it's the wrong desire? Gather your courage and butch up your act to make it true to your sexual personality. Even if you are less of a hit on the streets or in the bars, it's more than likely you'll meet the exact cute kid you want, and whom everyone used to think you were.

Another aspect of types is that they can get in the way of beginning new relationships. You may only go out with short, stocky Mediterranean guys with dark seraglio eyes, but now find you've met a lanky, blue-eyed WASP who won't leave you alone and who seems strangely more simpatico—and even attractive—than your usual type. Unless you're willing to break your rigid type mold, you're not going to find out if this man is a potential romance or even life-mate.

Then there's the question of race (see *Racism*). Even the most intelligent and liberal among us harbor unconscious fears and hatreds, which have been years in the making by those around us stupider and more bigoted; these can strongly influence our selection of sex partners. Be aware and remain open. Try dating someone the exact opposite of your usual type. You could be very pleasantly surprised. You might never again have a type.

VANILLA SEX

Like the ice cream of the same name, it's both popular and plain. Used by some in a merely descriptive way, and by others pejoratively, "vanilla" refers to a person whose sexual fantasies and actions are among the most socially approved both in the gay world and by those straights on its periphery. An emphasis on kissing and affection, and a healthy dose of sucking and fucking are the basic repertoire of those who are called vanilla. They like hygienic bodies clad in freshly laundered

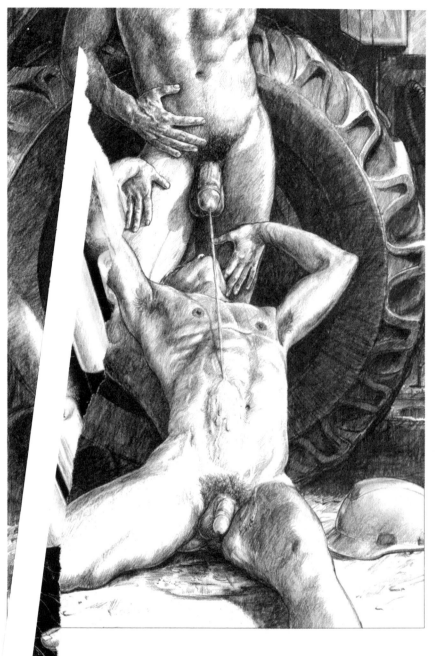

pes, and even forms of enema tube to be inserted inside them, as
vorite liquids to be squirted, from the simplest—warm water—to
ft drinks, their partner's piss, even expensive wines and fine co-
wever, using alcoholic drinks in large enough quantities (no one
w large) leads to quick absorption of the alcohol, which can
eath. Also be advised that excessive flushing of the colon may

WILLS

The ancient Egyptians were well prepared for death. They filled their tombs with furniture, food, jewelry, and all the things they thought would be needed in the afterlife. They believed they could "take it with them," an odd belief to us Westerners with our heads filled with fear over death and remorse over sin. We know we can't take it with us, and many of us worry about where we're going in our afterlife.

Thinking about wills is understandably distasteful to many men, because they don't like to think about dying. While giving lip service to the idea that we're all going to perish one way or another, we all secretly believe we're immortal and so we put off confronting death; to do so we use one or more rationalizations. The most common is "I don't have any money or property." You might not be a Donald Trump, but you would be surprised at how many things of value you possess. It might be worthwhile to go through your home and list what you own. Do this before making out a will, and along the way you might decide what to leave to various friends and family.

Even so, a will is not about money and things only. It's also about how you want to be remembered by family and friends. After all, it will probably be the only document that speaks for you after death, and that's especially important to gay people because we're seldom fully protected by law. Your wishes about your property, including items with sentimental value, and about the disposal of your body may not be respected if you don't have a will.

The HIV crisis has poignantly brought home the importance of will making. Some parents and family members are sympathetic to their gay sons and welcome their lovers in the family. Other parents, however, are spiteful, selfish people without the capacity for compassion or warmth, and they view their son's homosexuality as a blight upon their own reputation (see *Parents*). These parents often refuse to visit sons ill with HIV Disease, or to have contact with their son's lover. A gay man knows his situation and so he especially needs to protect both himself and his heirs, especially a lover or children, against parents like these. That's the function of a will.

When drawing up a will, a lawyer will ask for the following information:

1. A list of your valuables, including money and property.

2. A list of sentimental items.

3. How you want your body disposed of.

4. If you have minor children, who their guardians are to be.

5. Whom you want as executor of the estate.

In addition to these, quite a few gay men with HIV Disease have made special provisions in their wills. Holding a memorial service to celebrate one's life is one example. The will usually appoints a lover or friend to organize the service (it might even be a party!) and the estate provides the money to pay for it. This should be clearly stated in the will, which should also name those who are to do the work, and state the amount you wish to spend out of your estate.

You may want to discuss your will with your parents or family, but *only* if you have a good relationship with them. You might even want them to have a copy of the will. By doing so you'll put them on notice about your wishes. If you have a lover, you may want him to join in this discussion. It's also common for gay men who feel rejected by their primary families to think of their closest friends as their new family. They may look to these new family members when appointing executors and designating heirs. It may be wise to tell your parents or siblings that a friend, or your lover, or someone else you name will be your executor and that you've discussed your wishes with him or her in detail. On the other hand, be careful about disclosing too much information (or even any) if your parents disapprove of your gay life and are certain to cause problems after your death. These are questions that should be discussed with your attorney.

Can parents or siblings contest your will? Yes. Any will can be contested, but the fact is that 99 percent of the time the will you wrote stands up in court. It's just that you don't want your heirs to go through the hassle and additional legal fees. Traditionally a will can be contested in three ways:

1. It was improperly executed. Handwritten and quirky wills usually fall into this category. Any attorney who deals often with gay people will know how to write the will to conform to state law.

2. It was the result of undue influence. This used to be a favorite way for parents to contest a will by a gay son who left all or the bulk of his estate to a lover. The argument—no longer accepted in courts—is that the lover seduced the son and made him homosexual.

3. The gay man was incompetent to make out the will. This argument can be raised when a person is mentally or physically incapable of understanding the components of the will. In other words, make out your will when you're still in good contact with your mental faculties. Don't wait until you're in a coma.

Also note that when a person dies within a certain short period of time after making out a will—even a perfectly legitimate will—the state or municipal court (or an estate court) may hold it up for a thorough examination of the circumstances of the death. The time varies from state to state, but is usually under a year.

Your will is not the only way to protect a lover, children, and friends. Other ways include insurance policies, bank accounts, joint holdings of property, and putting money into noncontestable funds (see *Insurance; Living Wills*). Lovers need to discuss their joint holdings, and in discussion with legal advisors, arrange to protect themselves (and their children) in the event that one of them dies.

Be aware that any large property that you own only in your name and which you wish to will to someone else after your death will force your estate into a process called probate. This is literally "proving" the will: that is, your ownership of the property, its value, and all other aspects of your will. Houses, condos, cars, and bank accounts generally force probate, which can take from months to a year. Books have been written showing how to avoid this process. If the time factor is a concern for you and your legatees, look into this; you might want to make a bequest while you're still alive, or even "sell" the property for a minuscule amount of money.

WRESTLING

Many homosexuals like to wrestle before or even during sex. For some, wrestling is a virtual substitute for sex. Whereas some men like to know from the outset the role they will play during a particular sexual encounter, others are only truly excited when there's a struggle to determine who will be "top man," which is tantamount to saying who will do the fucking, and who will get fucked. Luckily, people have different tastes, and while winning may be thrilling, in wrestling defeat can be pleasurable too.

The pleasure is not only one of vying for position. It comes from the sensuality entailed when two strong male bodies engage in strenuous physical exertion: back muscles flare, biceps bulge, sweat flows, buttocks become rigid with strain. For some men the prevailing flat hardness of flesh, the rigid musculature, the long exposed bones that so totally contrast the male body to the female are the real turn-on. Allied (perhaps) to memories of adolescent or juvenile roughhouse play, such physical combativeness and competition, with its underlying threat of real harm and the possibility of total subjugation, can become the ultimate aphrodisiac.

Some given to wrestling have well-equipped game rooms with professional mats. The main difference between professional and sexual bouts, however, is that the latter are almost always done in the nude, or at most with the pair clad only in jockstraps. Often wrestlers oil their bodies. Climax is sometimes achieved through fucking and sucking, though some wrestlers like to end up in a clinch—jerking off. Wrestling can also be integrated into S/M sessions, with the difference that the master-slave question is decided not in advance but in action, right there on the mat.

INDEX

AA. *See* Alcoholics Anonymous
Abandonment, 66, 109, 124, 152, 162
Abuse, 56–57
  in childhood, 59–60, 125–26
ACOA. *See* Adult Children of Alcoholics
Acton, William, 119
ACT UP, 80, 82, 85, 163
  as macho style, 128, 130–31
Adolescence, *xiii*, 4, 34–35, 189, 190, 191–94, 202
Adoption, 26, 42, 82
Adult Children of Alcoholics (ACOA), 18
Affection, 53, 54. *See also* Love; Tenderness
African-Americans, 131, 152–53, 204, 207
Age, lying about, 140
Aging, older men, 42, 83–84. *See also* Daddy-son fantasies
AIDS (HIV Disease), *xv*, 2, 12–15, 25, 36, 44, 46, 66, 67, 80, 82, 85, 89–94, 106, 107, 114, 150, 153, 188, 192, 200, 212–13
  asymptomatic, 90
  condom use to prevent, 40, 41, 115
  contact tracing of, 27
  diagnosis of, 91
  and discrimination, 27
  and educational funding, 27
  insurance coverage for, 101, 102–3
  and mandatory testing, 27
  mixed couples, 124–25
  and opportunistic infections, 91, 93
  and oral sex, 10, 11
  parents of patients, *xv*, 14, 188–89, 212, 213

symptoms of, 91–92
  testing for, 90–91, 101
  transmission of, 72, 132, 156, 162, 163, 168, 185
AIDS Treatment News, 94
Air express, 188
Alacoque, Margaret Mary, 158
Al-Anon, 18
Alcoholics Anonymous, 18
Alcohol use and abuse, 16–18, 20, 29, 47, 57, 58, 59, 68, 71, 90, 97–98, 136, 141, 162, 175, 198, 211
Alexander the Great, 95
Alienation, 112, 145
Alyson Press, 42
Ambivalence, 199
Amebiasis, 156
American Model Guild, 148
American Psychiatric Association, *Diagnostic and Statistical Manual,* 120
Amphetamines, 16, 58
Amyl nitrate, 58
Anal intercourse, *xiv*, 1, 4, 7, 8, 11, 15, 26, 40, 41, 54, 72, 89, 108, 114, 127, 133, 142, ·144, 146, 148–49, 150, 156, 157, 161, 163, 168, 170, 172, 173, 175, 176, 177, 179–80, 186, 214
  first time, 67–71, 76. *See also* Sexual positions
Androgens, 126
Anglo macho image, 130–31
Anus, 1, 10, 62, 72, 76, 89, 156, 173, 174, 177, 179, 183
  relaxation exercises, 67–68
Anxiety, 116, 122, 149, 155, 156, 200
Aphrodisiacs, 171, 214
Approach-avoidance pattern, 96
Aretino, Pietro, *Postures,* 146

Aristophanes, 41–42
Aristotle, 126
Arms, 10
Arthritis, 173
Asian-Americans, 131, 153
Attachment, 42, 44
A-200 (drug), 175
Autoerotic asphyxiation, 52
Autonomy, 44
AZT, 94

Bacillary dysentery, 165
Back problems, 64
Back rooms, 190–91
Back Street, 116
Ball Park (Denver bathhouse), 2
Bankhead, Tallulah, 25
Barbiturates, 16, 97
Bars, 1–2, 3, 16–17, 29, 45, 47, 54, 76, 80, 84, 96, 141, 146, 152, 165, 208. *See also* Leather bars
Baths, 2–3, 146, 168
Battery. *See* Domestic violence; S/M
Bear (macho style), 87, 128, 130, 131, 208
Beards and mustaches, 87, 128, 130, 186, 208. *See also* Hair and shaving
Beauty, 3–4. *See also* Macho images; Types and typecasting
Beecher, Henry Ward, 146
Belly fucking, 76
Belts, 49, 169, 170
Benjamin, Harry, 204
Benkert, Karoly Maria, 78
Bestiality, 170–71
Biceps, 65, 214
Bijou, 146, 148
Bisexuality, 4, 6–8, 94–95, 127, 202

Biting. *See* Nibbling and biting
Bjorg, Kristin, 148
"Blind walk" game, 60
Blood, 11, 90
Blood tests, 172, 173, 174
Blow jobs, 7, 8–10, 11, 14, 15, 26,
    38, 40, 41, 54, 63, 70, 76, 89,
    133, 142, 144, 148, 149, 157,
    163, 168, 170, 173, 175, 176,
    181, 186, 200, 202, 210, 214.
    See also Sixty-nining
Body, as fetish, 65
Body fluids. *See* Blood; Saliva;
    Semen
Body image, 11–12, 145
Body positive. *See* AIDS (HIV
    Disease)
Body Positive (support group),
    13
Bondage, 15–16. *See also* S/M
Boredom, 122
Boston, domestic-partnership
    rights in, 27
Boswell, James, 38–39
Botel Gym, 86
Bottom position, 18–20, 56, 76,
    180, 183, 197, 210
Boys in the Sand, 146, 148
Breaking up, 109–10
Browning, Robert, 146
Bryant, Anita, *xiv*
Bullough, Vern, 171
Buns (buttocks), 130, 180, 200
    as erogenous zone, 2, 12, 18, 20–
    22, 89, 132, 214
    exercises for, 21–22
    as fetish, 65, 146. *See also* Anal
    intercourse; Spanking
Burton, Richard, 72, 171
"Butch"/"femme" roles, 197–98.
    See also "Masculine" and
    "feminine" roles; Types and
    typecasting
Butt plugs, 170
Butyl nitrate, 58

Camping, 23–25, 61
Canada, *Joy* publishing history, *xiv*
Cancer, 93, 101
Carding, 152–53
Cardiovascular syphilis, 174
Carpenter, Edward, 78
Castration, 127, 128
Catholic church, 25
    sadomasochism in, 158
Cat-litter-box filler, 93
Cauldwell (sexologist), 204
Ceftriaxone, 173
Celibacy, 25
Censorship, *xiv, xvi*
Centers for Disease Control, 91, 189
Chains, 169
Chastity belts, 170
"Chatting," in computer sex, 37

Child custody cases, 82
Child molestation, 59–60, 125–26,
    181, 192
Children, 115, 116, 212, 214
China, 171, 174
Chippendale's, 128
Chlamydia, 177
Circumcision, 72–74
Civil rights, *xiii*, 2, 26–27, 36, 82,
    85. *See also* Gay liberation,
    gay militancy
Clap. *See* Gonorrhea
Clap, Margaret, 172
Cleanliness, excessive, 85
Cleopatra, 8
Clothing, 46, 49. *See also* Leather;
    Macho images
Clubs, 27–30, 45, 76, 80, 133, 141,
    146, 152, 162, 165. *See also*
    J.O. clubs
Club 7009 (Beverly Hills
    bathhouse), 2
CMV. *See* Cytomegalovirus
COBRA law, 102
Cocaine, 16, 57, 58, 59
Cock enlargement pumps, 30, 169–
    70
Cock rings, 99, 100, 169
Cogan, Thomas, 123
Coitus interruptus, 170
Cold sores, 93, 176
Colette, 87
Colorado, AIDS discrimination in,
    27
Colostomy, 71
Columbus, Christopher, 174
Coming out, *xv*, 32–36, 37–39, 192,
    194
Compulsion to please, 85
Compulsive behavior, 85
Compulsive sex, 150–51, 152, 207
Computer sex, 36–38, 48
Condoms, 2, 10, 11, 38–41, 52, 62,
    68, 114, 115, 136, 161, 163,
    164, 168, 172
Consensual acts, 84–85
Cornholing. *See* Anal intercourse
Costumes, 122. *See also* Leather
Couples, 41–45, 110
Covenant House, 194
Crabs, 172, 175
Crack, 58, 59
Crisco, 40, 114
Cronkite, Walter, 140
Cruising, *xiii*, 2, 11, 45–48, 84, 85,
    96
Cryptococcal meningitis, 93
Crystal, 58
"Cut" vs. "uncut" meat, 73, 140
Cytomegalovirus (CMV), 13, 93

Daddy-son fantasies, 48–50, 87,
    179, 187, 192, 208
Daddy: The Magazine, 50

Dancing, 29, 58
Dashwood, Francis, 160
Date rape, 153
Daughters of Bilitis, 79
DDI (drug), 94
Death and grieving, *xv,* 12, 53,
    110–11, 113, 139, 162, 176,
    211
Deltoids, 65
Dementia, 93
DeMille, Cecil B., 135
Dental dams, 157
Depression, *xiii*, 12, 53–54, 85, 93,
    109, 112, 155, 188
    learned, 53
    as repressed anger, 53
Desensitization, 149
Diabetes, 99
Different Light Bookstore, 137
Dildos, 52, 68, 161, 169, 170, 210
Dirty talk, 10, 54–55, 105, 161
Discrimination. *See* Civil rights
Disinhibition, 17
Divorce, 26
"Docking," 73
Dog collars, 170
Doggy style, 55–56
Domestic partnerships, domestic-
    partnership rights, 26–27, 42,
    102
Domestic violence, *xv,* 56–57
Domination, 15, 71, 74, 183. *See
    also* S/M
Downs. *See* Barbiturates
Drag. *See* Transvestism
Drug contouring, 57, 58
Drug use and abuse, 16–18, 20, 29,
    57–59, 68, 71, 90, 97–98, 136,
    141, 160, 162, 163, 175, 178,
    192, 198. *See also* specific
    drugs
Drummer, 145

Earrings, 131, 144. *See also*
    Piercing
Eastern Europe, 78, 189
EBV. *See* Epstein-Barr virus
Ecstasy, 58, 141
Effeminacy, 61, 95, 197–98. *See
    also* "Masculine" and
    "feminine" roles; Types and
    typecasting
Egypt (ancient), 119, 212
Eight-Plus Club, 107
Ejaculation problems, 150–52, 169,
    177
Emphysema, 173
Endorphins, 145
Enemas, 1, 68, 163, 210–11
England. *See* United Kingdom
Entamoeba Histolytica, 176
Envy, 104
Eon de Beaumont, Chevalier d',
    203

Epstein-Barr virus (EBV), 13, 93
Erectile-dysfunction clinics, 98–99, 100
Escort services, 96, 97
Estrogens, 126
Exploitation, 162, 192

Face-to-face position, 56, 61–64
Family, 12, 35. *See also* Coming out; Marriage; Parents
Fantasies, 25, 37, 41, 96, 97, 100, 105–6, 140, 148, 150, 154, 158, 160, 166, 187
masturbation and, 119–23
Fatigue, 175
Fears, 149
Feces, 1, 11, 164–65, 173, 175, 176–77
Fellatio. *See* Blow jobs; Sixty-nining
Feminism, feminists, 24, 146, 153
Fetishism, 64–65
Fever, 92, 175
FFA. *See* Fistfuckers of America
Fidelity and monogamy, 44, 65–66, 150. *See also* Infidelity
Filthy, 148
Fire Island Pines, 58, 86, 136
Fistfuckers of America (FFA), 71, 160
Fisting, 71–72, 114, 160, 163
Fists of Fury, 71
Flagellation, 158
Flirting, 153, 165
Foot fetishism, 64, 65
Foreskin, 73, 172
ForPlay (lubricant), 40, 114
Fort Lauderdale, 86
France, *xiv,* 38, 171, 174
Frederick the Great, 171
Freedom of association, 80, 81
Free speech, 14
French kissing, 11, 107. *See also* Kissing
Frenum piercing, 144
Freud, Sigmund, 4, 94
Oedipus complex and homosexuality, 127
Fricke, Aaron, *Reflections of a Rock Lobster,* 192
Friends and lovers, *xiii,* 18, 35, 36, 48, 54, 57, 74, 109–10, 112, 117, 138, 150, 152, 163, 165, 188
of AIDS patients, 12, 13, 14, 124–25, 212–13
Frottage, 74, 76
Fuck buddies, 68, 76, 117

GAA. *See* Gay Activists Alliance
Gage, Joe, 148
Gag response, 8
Gags, 170
Ganymede Press, 50

Garland, Judy, 203
Gauntlet, Inc., 145
Gay Activists Alliance (GAA), 79–80
Gay and Lesbian Alliance Against Discrimination, (GLAAD), 80
Gay bars. *See* Bars
Gay-bashing, 153
Gay bookstores, 2
GayCom (computer network), 38
Gayellow Pages, 1, 67
Gay health services, 67, 80
Gay liberation, gay militancy, 29, 65, 67, 78–80, 81, 97, 103, 197, 198, 202
Gay Liberation Front, 79, 80
Gay magazines and newspapers, 89, 96, 139, 162. *See also* Pornography; *specific titles*
Gay Men's Health Crisis (GMHC), 94
Gay politics and politicians, 80–83
Gay rights, 81, 103
Gay stereotypes, 61, 95, 128–31. *See also* Types and Typecasting
Georgia: sodomy law in, 81
Germany, 78, 144
Giardia lamblia, 176
GLAAD. *See* Gay and Lesbian Alliance Against Discrimination
Glad Day Bookshops, *xiv*
Gluteus maximus, 21–22. *See also* Buns (buttocks)
GMHC. *See* Gay Men's Health Crisis
Gold's Gym, 86
Gonorrhea, 39, 156, 172–73, 177
Gordon, Charles George, 95
Graham, Sylvester, 119
Granger, Thomas, 170–71
Greece (ancient), 4
Guiche, 144
Guilt feelings, 13, 17, 48, 84–85, 96, 103–4, 116, 124, 145, 149, 151, 184
Guppie (gay yuppie) macho style, 128, 130, 131
Gyms, 86, 114

Hair and shaving, 2, 12, 49, 87, 178–79
Hairbrushes, 49
Hairy leukoplakia, 92
Hallucinogens, 68
Halstead, Fred, 148
Handcuffs, 169
Handkerchief, as S/M signal, 160
Hands, 8–9, 10, 12, 49, 88–89, 109, 176, 199
Harvey Milk School, 191
Hashish, 58
Hawkins, Ronald, *xiv*

Hays, Harry, 79
Heart disease, 101
Hebrews (ancient), 72
Hedwig, Sophia, 204
Hell Fire Club, 160
Hepatitis, 13, 66–67, 90, 156, 165, 172, 175–76
Heroin, 58, 59
Herpes simplex, 13, 172, 176
Herpes viruses, 13, 92, 93–94
Hickeys, 131–32. *See also* Kissing
Hirschfeld, Magnus, 78, 203
HIV. *See* AIDS (HIV Disease)
Holleran, Andrew, *Dancer from the Fire,* 181
Hollywood film industry, 81
Homophobia, *xiii–xiv,* 10, 14, 16, 23, 24, 27, 36, 37, 42, 50, 53, 57, 59, 60, 61, 67, 81, 85, 94–96, 172, 189, 204
internalized, 85, 95–96, 202, 205
theories of, 94–96
Homosexuality, homosexuals. *See also Gay entries*
as genuine society and institution, 7
mythic origins of, 125–28
as parents, 82, 115, 116, 212, 214
and self-hatred, 145
Hormones, 30
Hustlers, 96–97, 108, 151, 194, 202, 204

Identification, 53
Immigration, 27
Impotence, 97–100, 149, 169
Industrial Revolution, 39
Infidelity, 65–66, 85, 103–4, 150. *See also* Fidelity and monogamy
Institute for Sexual Science, 78
Insurance, *xv,* 26, 101–3, 125, 205, 213
Interfemoral fucking, 76
Internal bleeding, 71
International Male, 146
Intimacy, 45, 54, 106, 108, 113–14, 142, 148, 188. *See also* Love
Intravenous needles, 163
Isay, Richard, *Being Homosexual: Gay Men and Their Development,* 48–49
Isherwood, Christopher, *Christopher and His Kind,* 78
Italy, 38, 174

Jacks (club), 107
Jacobus. *See* Sutor, Jacobus
James, Henry, 146
James, John S., 94
James, William, *The Varieties of Religious Experience,* 113
Jealousy, 66, 103–5
Jewelry. *See* Earrings; Piercing

Jews, 72
Joan of Arc, 202
J.O. buddies, 105–6, 114, 122
Jockstraps, 64, 65, 105, 136, 185, 214
J.O. clubs, *xv,* 106–7, 122, 168, 170
Johnson, Samuel, 38
Julius Caesar, 95, 142

Kaposi's Sarcoma (KS), 93
Karl, Herman, 204
Kellogg, John Harvey, 119
Keys, as S/M signal, 160
Key West, 58
Kinsey Report, 79, 191
Kissing, *xiv–xv,* 20, 56, 61, 63, 71, 88, 107–9, 131–32, 163, 173, 175, 181
Kitchener, Horatio, 95
Klein, Calvin, 128
Kwell, 175, 177
K-Y, 40, 114, 122

Ladder, The, 79
Laguna Beach, 86
Lambda Rising Bookstores, 137
Laser treatment, for venereal warts, 178
Latinos, 131, 152–53, 203
L.A. Tool & Die, 71
Lauren, Ralph, 128, 130
Leashes, 170
Leather, 1, 15, 38, 64, 87, 128
Leather bars, 130, 158, 159
Legs, 10, 65, 89, 105
Lenin, V. I., 130
Lesbianism, lesbians, 41, 80, 95, 126, 145, 191, 194, 197
Letting go, 109–11
Lew, Mike, *Victims No Longer,* 154
Lewis, Mrs. (condom monopoly holder), 38
Living wills, 111–12, 125
Loneliness, *xiii,* 112–14
Louis XIV, 203
Love, 3, 41–45, 57, 74, 97, 100, 103–4, 114, 142, 145, 154
and letting go, 109–11
and possessiveness, 65
Lovers. *See* Friends and lovers
Lubricants, 1, 38, 62, 68, 72, 76, 114–15, 136, 161, 179, 181. *See also* Saliva; specific lubricants
"Lurking," in computer sex, 37
Lymph nodes, 92, 174

MacDonald, Boyd, 148
Macho images, *xvi,* 87, 105, 128–31. *See also* Types and typecasting
McMaster University, *xiv*
Mafia, 16

Mandrax, 58
Mantegazza, Paolo, 171
Mardi Gras, 203
Mariages blancs, 44
Marijuana, 58, 97
Marlboro Man, 128
Marriage, 114, 115–16, 190
Martyr syndrome,145
Marvel Comics, 82
"Masculine" and "feminine" roles, 4, 6, 8, 20, 61, 157, 197–98. *See also* Types and typecasting
Massage, 117–18, 163
Master/slave relationship, 15, 20. *See also* Domination; Sex toys; S/M
Masturbation, 20, 25, 35, 38, 40, 41, 52, 56, 63, 65, 68, 70, 76, 105, 114, 127, 133, 135, 136, 144,'148, 149, 151, 154, 161, 163, 169, 170, 178, 180, 181, 188, 214
devices to prevent, 119
as "disorder," 120
and fantasy, 119–20
as "perversion," 120
on phone, 139, 140–41, 142
by women, 119–20
Mattachine Society, 79
Maya Indians, 142, 144
MDA (designer drug), 58
Meat, 148
Meat, undercooked, 93
Media, 80, 81, 85
Medicaid, 103
Memory problems, 93
Merrill's Gym, 86
Methedrine, 58
Michelangelo, *David,* 21
Mid-City Gym, 86
Mineshaft (NYC bar), 15–16
Mirrors, 20, 123–24, 178
Moldenhauer, Jearld, *xiv*
Motorcycle-club insignia, as S/M signal, 160
Mouth, 88, 108–9, 172, 174, 199. *See also* Kissing
Music, as aphrodisiac, 122, 136, 166
Muslims, 72

NA. *See* Narcotics Anonymous
Nar-Anon, 18
Narcissism, healthy, 124
Narcotics Anonymous (NA), 18
National Gay Task Force, 80
National Geographic, 146
Native Americans, 174
Nazis, 78
Neck stiffness, 93
Nembutal, 58–59
New Guinea, 125

New York City, 197
domestic-partnership rights in, 27
gay ghetto in, 197
"tearooms," in, 190
New York City Gay and Lesbian Anti-Violence Project, 154
New York City Marriage License Bureau, 80
New York State health-care proxy law, 111
New York Times, The, 57
Nibbling and biting, 109, 131–32, 188
Night sweats, 92
Nipple clamps, 133, 161, 170
Nipple rings, 134, 142, 144, 170. *See also* Piercing
Nipples, 10, 88, 109, 132–34, 181, 188
Nocturnal emissions, 25
Noisemaking, 134–35
Nonoxyl-9 spermicide, 40, 68, 114
Northstar (comic-book hero), 82
Nostalgie de la boue, 186

Obsessive love, 109–10
Obsessive sex. *See* Compulsive sex
One, 79
One-night stands, 44, 165, 206–7
On Our Backs, 145
Opportunistic infections, 91, 93
Oral sex. *See* Blow jobs; Sixty-nining
Orgies, 38, 135–36, 168
Orwell, George, *1984,* 109
Osiris, 119
"Outing," 92
Oxford University presses, 146

Paraphilias, 52, 165
Parasites, parasitic diseases, 66–67, 156, 165, 172, 176–77
Parents, 45, 74, 85, 116
of AIDS patients, *xv,* 14, 138–39, 212, 213
coming out to, 137–39
rejection by, 53, 205–6
revenge of, 61
supportiveness of, *xv,* 35
Parents and Friends of Lesbians and Gays (PFLAG), 137
Paresis, 174
Paris Is Burning, 203
Party drugs. *See* Hallucinogens
Passiveness and submission, 20, 54, 61–62, 154, 157, 186–87, 200
Pausanias, 78
Pazzi, Mary-Magdalen dei, 158
PCP. *See* Pneumocystis carinii pneumonia

PCP (designer drug), 58
Pectorals, 132, 146
Pederasty, 4. *See also* Child
  molestation
Peer pressure, 162
Penicillin, 174
Penile implants, 99–100
Penis, 1, 18, 88, 164, 172, 173, 174,
  176, 177, 180. *See also* Anal
  intercourse; Blow jobs;
  Masturbation; Sixty-nining
  piercing of, 144–45
  size of, 30, 32, 140, 146
People with Aids Coalition
  (PWAC), 23, 80, 94
Pericarditis, 173
Perineum, 71, 144
Peritonitis, 71
Persia, 127
Personal ads, *xv,* 18, 73, 136, 167–
  68
PFLAG. *See* Parents and Friends
  of Lesbians and Gays
Pheromones, 185
Phillips, Mrs. (condom monopoly
  holder), 38
Phimosis, 73
Phone sex, *xv,* 105, 139–42, 151
Physicians, 66–67, 100, 101–2, 111,
  188. *See also* Sexually
  transmitted diseases
Picano, Felice, *xii, xv*
Piercing, 52, 73, 131, 132, 142–45,
  210
Pissing. *See* Water sports
Plato, *Symposium,* 41–42, 78
Pleasure, pleasure problems, 117–
  18, 120, 145, 200
Pleasure Chest, 41
Pneumocystis carinii pneumonia
  (PCP), 92–93
Police, 16, 17, 80, 154, 190
Politeness, excessive, 85
Political activism, political
  awareness, *xv,* 29, 36. *See
  also* Gay liberation, gay
  militancy
Pornography, 3, 34, 41, 48, 120,
  122, 124, 146–48, 150, 158,
  166, 186, 187. *See also
  individual titles*
Possessiveness, 65, 195
Precome, 10, 11, 40, 41. *See also*
  Semen
Prejudice. *See* Homophobia
Prenatal theory of homosexuality,
  126–27
Prepuce, 73. *See also* Foreskin;
  Piercing
Prince Albert piercing, 144
Princeton rub, 76
Prisons, imprisonment, 128, 154
Progressive relaxation, 156
Project Inform, 94

Promiscuity, 150–52. *See also*
  One-night stands
Prostate gland, 1, 71, 177, 183
Prostatitis, 172, 177
Prostitutes. *See* Hustlers
Proust, Marcel, *Remembrance of
  Things Past,* 103
Provincetown, 58
Psychoanalysis, 127
Psychotherapy, 18, 25, 50, 54, 60,
  85, 98, 100, 110–11, 116, 145,
  150, 152, 155, 165, 188
Public toilets. *See* Tearooms
Pumping Iron, 86
"Pump Nights," 170
Putassa, La, 203
PWAC. *See* People with Aids
  Coalition
PWAC Newsline, 94

Quääludes, 58
Queer Nation, 80, 85, 163
Quick sex, 114

Racism, *xv,* 152–53, 207, 208
Racks, 170
Rage, Christopher, 148
Rape, *xv,* 153–54
  fantasies of, 154
  by father or stepfather, 154
Rape crisis lines, 154
Ratner, Ellen, *The Other Side of
  the Family: A Book for
  Recovering from Abuse,* 60
Reaper (paraphilia), 52
Recruitment theory of
  homosexuality, 125–26
Rectum. *See* Anus
Rejection, *xiii,* 13, 17, 53, 54, 139,
  155, 189
Relaxation, 156
Relaxation exercises, 67–68
Renaissance House, 67
Rid, 175
Right wingers, 146
Rimming, 62, 156–57, 163, 165,
  175, 176, 180–81, 184, 200
Ritch Street Baths, 2
Roberto/Roberta, 203
Role playing, 157–58. *See also*
  Types and typecasting
Roller dancers, 30
Roman Empire, 4, 72
Romano, Giulio, 146
Ropes, 161
Rough sex, 89, 202. *See also* S/M
Rubber (designer drug), 58
Rubber, as fetish, 96

Sacher-Masoch, Leopold von, 158
Sade, Donatien Alphonse, Marquis
  de, *120 Days of Sodom,* 158
Sadomasochism. *See* S/M
Safe word, in S/M, 160

SAGE. *See* Senior Action in a Gay
  Environment
Saliva, 8–9, 11, 13, 62, 132, 180,
  181, 200
Samaritans, 189
San Francisco
  domestic-partnership rights in,
  26–27
  gay ghetto in, 197
Sappho, 44
Saran Wrap, 157
Saying no, 163–64, 210. *See also*
  Rejection
Scabies, 172, 177
Scat. *See* Feces
Scenes, 158
Schwarzenegger, Arnold, 37
Scoppetone, Sandra, *Trying Hard
  to Hear You,* 192
Scrotum, 10
SeaHorse Press, *xii*
Seattle, domestic-partnership
  rights in, 27
Seborrheic dermatitis, 72
Seconal, 58–59
Seduction, 165–66
Self-acceptance, self-esteem, 1,
  3–4, 13, 25, 35, 53, 59, 104–5,
  145, 162, 192
  and body image, 11–12
Self-contempt, self-hatred, 85, 95–
  96, 145
Self-pity, 155
Semen, 11, 13, 25, 40, 90, 163, 175,
  177, 185, 186
Senior Action in a Gay
  Environment (SAGE), 84
Serial monogamy, 150
Service organizations, 67, 85, 88,
  89, 94, 102, 163. *See also*
  Support groups
Sex, 53–54, 58
  dangerous, unsafe, *xv, xvi,* 2, 15,
  17, 50, 52, 59, 72, 97, 107, 151,
  156, 168, 171, 186
  nonconsensual, *xiv*
  safe, *xv, xvi,* 3, 13–14, 18,
  20, 44, 46–47, 94, 106, 149,
  150, 161–63, 185, 186, 192,
  207
  "sleazy," *xvi,* 184–86, 210
  "vanilla," *xvi,* 208, 210
Sex ads. *See* Personal ads
Sex clubs, 2–3, 168. *See also* J.O.
  clubs
Sexology, 204
Sex therapy, 117, 150
Sex toys, 30, 52, 151, 161, 163,
  169–70, 210
  condoms as, 39
Sexually transmitted diseases
  (STDs), *xiii,* 13–14, 38–39, 66–
  67, 107, 154, 172–78. *See also*
  specific diseases

Sexual positions
  bottoms up, 20
  doggy style, 55–56
  face-to-face, 56
  side-by-side, 52, 149, 179–80
  sitting on it, 149, 181–83
  standing, 187–88
Sex with animals. *See* Bestiality
Shakespeare, William, *Hamlet,* 186
Shingles, 92, 93
Shit. *See* Feces
Shock treatment, 128
Side-by-side position, 56, 149, 179–80
Sigmoid colon, 71, 72
Silverstein, Charles, *xii–xiii, xiv, xv*
  Man to Man: Gay Couples in America, 44, 48
  and White, Edmund, *The Joy of Gay Sex, xi–xii, xiii–xv*
"Simon Says" game, 60
Simultaneous orgasm, 63
Sitting on it position, 149, 181–83
Sixty-nining, 8, 26, 108, 157, 183–84. *See also* Blow jobs
Sleeping pills, 58–59
Slim disease, 92
Slings, 170
S/M, 15, 20, 71, 85, 106, 133, 144–45, 158–61, 163, 164, 169, 170, 210, 214
Smut, 148
Society for Human Rights, 79
Sodomy, sodomy laws, 26, 81, 170
Sontag, Susan, "Notes on Camp," 24
Soviet Union, 78
Spanking, 49, 63, 186–87, 210
Special K (designer drug), 58
Standing position, 187–88
STAR. *See* Street Transvestite Activist Revolutionaries
Starlight Express, 30
Stereotypes. *See* Types and typecasting
Steroids, 86
Stockades, 170
Stomach, 10, 65, 128
Stonewall riot, 27, 40, 79, 80, 197, 198, 202, 204
Street Transvestite Activist Revolutionaries (STAR), 204
Streisand, Barbra, 203
Suicidal feelings, 53, 102, 188–89
Support groups, 13, 42, 60, 111, 116, 154, 189, 191. *See also specific groups*
Sutor, Jacobus, 30
Sweat, as aphrodisiac, 185, 186

Symonds, J. A., 78
Syphilis, 14, 94, 156, 172, 173–74

Tanizaki, Junichiro:
  The Secret History of the Lord of Musashi, 65
  Seven Japanese Tales, 65
Tardieu, A. (French physician), 126
Tattoos, 144
T-cells, 17, 91
Tearooms, 17, 48, 189–91
Teenagers. *See* Adolescence
Tenderness, 194–95
Testicles, 10, 86, 88, 132, 170, 177, 178, 179, 180
  piercing of, 144
Three-way, 188, 190, 195–97
Thrush, 92
Tissot (French physician), 119
Tool Chest, 41
Top position, 18, 76, 141–42, 183, 197–98, 210, 214
Touching and holding, 14–15, 54, 60, 186, 199–200
Toxoplasmosis, 93
Trade, 202. *See also* S/M
Transsexualism, transsexuals, 203, 204–5
Transvestism, transvestites, 27, 29, 178, 202–4
Treatment Issues, 94
Tricks, tricking, 15, 17, 36, 50, 52, 54, 66, 87, 112, 151, 154, 156, 160, 163, 205–7
Triggers, 60
Trucks (NYC area), 24
Trust, 60, 71
Tuinal, 58–59
Turkey, 174
Types and typecasting, *xvi,* 2, 3, 47, 54, 61, 96, 104, 115–16, 119–20, 128–31, 197–98, 207–8

Ulrichs, Karl, 78
"Uniform," 46
United Kindgom
  condom history in, 38–39
  Joy publishing history, *xiv*
  treatment of homosexuals in, 78
United States. *See also* U.S. Congress; U.S. Supreme Court; *individual states and cities*
  circumcision in, 72
  gay rights movement in, 79–80
  sex with animals in, 171
  treatment of homosexuals in, 78–80

Unrequited love, 109–10
Urethra, 10, 40, 52, 144, 172, 177
Urethritis, 172, 177
Urine, 173, 175, 177, 185, 186, 210. *See also* Water sports
"Urning," 78
U.S. Congress, 27
  gay members of, 82
U.S. Patent Office, antimasturbation devices, 119
U.S. Postal Service, 79
U.S. Supreme Court, 26, 79, 81

Vagina dentata theory of homosexuality, 126, 127
Vaseline, 40, 114, 122
Vastation, 113
Venereal diseases. *See* Sexually transmitted diseases (STDs)
Venereal warts, 172, 177–78
Venus, 172
Vibrators, 169
Violence, 89, 160. *See also* S/M
Virgil, *xvi,* 38
Voice, as erotic stimulus, 139–40, 142
Volunteer work. *See* Service organizations

Wall Street Shark macho style, 128, 130, 131
Water sports, 87, 163, 210–11
Weight loss, 92
West, Mae, 20
West Hollywood
  domestic-partnership rights in, 27
  gay government in, 81
Whips, 169
White, Edmund, *xv*
Wilde, Oscar, 78
Wills, *xv,* 82, 102, 112, 125, 139, 212–14. *See also* Living wills
Women
  clothing of, as fetish, 65
  insulted by camping, 24
  masturbation by, 119–20
  roles of, 95
Wordsworth, William, 59
Workaholism, 85
Work problems, 17
World League for Sexual Reform, 78
World War I, 144
World War II, 39, 42, 78, 79
Wrestling, 214

Young, Ian, 133

"Zapping," 80

ABOUT THE AUTHORS

Dr. Charles Silverstein is a clinical psychologist and psychotherapist who practices in New York City. He founded two counseling centers for gay people, the Institute for Human Identity and Identity House. He is also the founding editor of the *Journal of Homosexuality*. He was the psychologist who, in 1973, made the presentation before the Nomenclature Committee of the American Psychiatric Association that ultimately led to the removal of homosexuality from the list of mental disorders. The American Psychological Association honored him for his psychological work with the gay community by elevating him to the status of Fellow of the association.

Felice Picano is the author of twelve books—novels, short stories, poetry, translated into six languages—among them *The Lure, Late in the Season, Ambidextrous,* and *Men Who Loved Me*. He's also written reviews, essays, and screenplays and has had two plays produced off-Broadway. As founder and publisher of SeaHorse Press and cofounder of Gay Presses of New York, he's responsible for introducing the work of Harvey Fierstein, Doric Wilson, Dennis Cooper, Brad Gooch, Alan Bowne, and many other writers.

ABOUT THE ARTISTS

Deni Ponty was born and raised in the Netherlands, where he attended the Royal Academy of Fine and Applied Arts in the Hague. He continued his studies in the United States at several art colleges, and his work is now in collections around the world. A collection of his art, *Intimate Angel,* was published by GMP, London. He now lives and works in his studio in Los Angeles.

A native of the South, artist/illustrator *F. Ronald Fowler* received his Bachelor of Fine Arts from Pratt Institute in Brooklyn. Fowler's work has been seen in the New York City Society of Illustrators, on more than thirty book jackets, in men's magazines, and in the famous Provincetown Carnival Poster Series, and is represented in numerous public and private collections.